A LIFE WITHOUT MIGRAINES

To Laura,

thanks for being
who I created this
clinic for! My ideal
client!

A LIFE WITHOUT MIGRAINES

A HOLISTIC AND LITTLE-KNOWN METHOD FOR LIVING A HEADACHE-FREE LIFE

DR. GRANT DENNIS

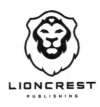

LIONCREST

PUBLISHING

A LIFE WITHOUT MIGRAINES

A Holistic and Little-Known Method For
Living a Headache-Free Life

ISBN   978-1-5445-1454-3   *Hardcover*

978-1-5445-1453-6   *Paperback*

978-1-5445-1452-9   *Ebook*

*To all those who have suffered and no longer must
live in suffering, and to those giants who came before
me and paved the way for healing to occur.*

CONTENTS

———

FOREWORD

———

During the last twenty-five years, I have sat in the waiting rooms of many doctors. I was always in pain. Years ago, I had a spinal surgery, hoping I would be healed for the rest of my life, but relief was only temporary. In the years following, I had many painful flare-ups that seemed to come at the most inconvenient times. I tried family doctors, neurologists, orthopedists, physical therapists, and several chiropractors. At each appointment, I would wait for long periods of time, my anxiety level rising every minute. I would wonder, "Is this just another disappointing effort to become pain-free? Will anything ever stop this head and neck pain?"

I was exhausted on many levels, and my life had become more and more limited. A friend told me about a chiropractor who provided healing through a unique kind of treatment. I researched Dr. Grant Dennis in Little Rock, Arkansas, and found that his knowledge, training, and experience met every qualification. I had doubts, but my friend was pain-free and I was not, so I called for the free diagnostic consultation that the doctor offered.

As I walked into his office, I began to experience something I had never felt before in a doctor's office. At first, it felt as if a fresh spring breeze was blowing through. I looked at the words written in calligraphy on one wall. They read, "They shall lay hands on them and they will get well" (Mark 16:18).

At that point, I knew there was not really a fresh spring breeze, but what I was experiencing was hope! I had forgotten. *Hope*. As Dr. Dennis and I discussed my case, I realized that I was face-to-face with *kindness*! He did not rush me through the appointment and quickly escort me out. I realized he wanted me to get well. He was dedicated and fully qualified, and he knew I was a good candidate.

At that point in my life, I was desperate to begin living a full life again. I was tired of feeling like a burden in my home. I wanted to do my part! I wanted to travel to see my children and grandchildren. I wanted to work more. I wanted to be able to write without pain striking my head and back. I wanted my full life again.

When my radiology report came back, Dr. Dennis and I discussed my condition. He said, "You are a perfect fit for the treatment I offer. You will soon be doing things that you never thought you would ever do again!"

I thought, "Could this possibly really be true? Do I dare enter into this healing process and let myself believe that?" I had been disappointed so many times, but as Dr. Dennis explained the treatment and expressed confidence and encouragement, I began to believe...and I got better. And better. And better.

Six months have passed since that first day. I just made two trips to see my children and grandchildren. I am working more. I am writing right now with no pain. My husband is thrilled to see a wife who can look forward to a new life, rather than being stuck in pain and getting worse as I age. Everything Dr. Dennis promised has happened!

In his quiet, comforting resting room, listening to soft music and the small rippling fountain before and after adjustments, I have heard similar stories from many people. I have not heard one negative word or any disappointment. Each person has commented on the expertise and kindness of Dr. Dennis, as well as his dedication to the healing of every one of his patients. And like me, they are getting better and better, with ALL kinds of different conditions.

The treatment is amazing, as are the results! I know

that I was given the opportunity to join in a healing process that also called for my dedication to a schedule of appointments. I no longer felt helpless. I began to see that my efforts were working. I looked forward to my appointments because I knew that gradually I would—and will—recover. I knew that I was in the finest hands, and I am so thankful that my life has been returned to me.

I would refer anyone who is in pain to try a free consultation with Dr. Grant Dennis. If you are a candidate for his treatment program, your life will never be the same!

Lynda D. Elliott
Author, life coach, and former social worker

INTRODUCTION

―――

This invisible disease has haunted me my entire life—like a ghost in the night—

It has haunted me so long that I wonder:

Am I losing my mind?

Nobody believes me.

I feel alone and find solace only in isolation.

I miss life events because of this ghost.

I feel guilt and regret even though I am powerless against it.

I am mentally exhausted and not sure how much longer I can live like this.

My quality of life is pathetic—

as if I have a disability that can't be seen by the human eye.

I am a migraine sufferer.

This is the everyday self-talk and reflection that occurs in the mind of a chronic migraine sufferer. If you are reading this, then you or someone dear to you is more than likely a sufferer, and it is all too familiar.

There is no worse feeling of weakness and powerlessness than suffering from a disease, and yes, migraines are a disease. However, they yield normal MRIs, normal lab findings, normal *everything*.

Yet, things are definitely not normal in your head—or in your life.

I always say until you've had head pain so severe that you are willing to do literally anything—and I mean *anything*—to make it subside, you have not experienced a migraine.

Migraines make you wake up wondering what the day will hold and praying heavily that one won't leave you just trying to survive until day's end.

A migraine is like a storm that is creeping in: you see it

coming, you feel it coming, and then when it rains, it literally pours, and there is no shelter for you to get under.

It starts as a dull throb in the back of the head or neck, and then progressively as the day goes on, it gets worse and worse, creeping up on you slowly.

You think to yourself, "Here it comes..."

It leaves you anxious, scared, and begging not to progress into a full-blown hurricane that will leave you riding out the storm like a small boat lost at sea, just hoping not to capsize over the next twenty-four to seventy-two hours.

It gets to the point where you constantly have to plan your entire life around the possibility of a migraine hitting, and the entire day is over.

Missed days of work, missed nights out with friends— you get to where you miss out on all the fun and exciting things in life because of migraines, and not one single doctor can find anything wrong with you.

This disease ends marriages and other relationships, ends jobs, ends careers, and affects the quality of lives.

Sound familiar?

What if I told you that you and your fellow migraine suf-ferers were looking for all the wrong things, in all the wrong places?

What if I told you the potential root cause of your problem could actually be VERY evident and obvious to a doctor who knew where to look? What if I told you that cause has been proven to explain a large majority of migraine cases that don't respond to traditional Western medicine routes?

At this point, you're probably beginning to think you are a "doctor's worst nightmare."

If you feel this way, even subconsciously, then I have good news for you. There's a doctor out there who will not consider you a nightmare. In fact, you are likely their ideal client!

There is a doctor who can meet you where you are and explain to you that your disease is real and indeed has a real cause. We locate the cause in helping people remove migraines from their life every day, and we help people like you every single day.

Sadly, there is not enough awareness among migraine sufferers, and there certainly are not enough holistic, natural, root-cause-eliminating, viable options out there in the world for these people!

While you might feel like you are alone, you are not alone. The feeling you get when you finally find a doctor who listens to you, believes in your ability to heal, and will partner with you every step of the way is exhilarating and empowering.

While you search for answers, there is a population of doctors searching for you!

I'm Dr. Grant Dennis, and I, too, was a migraine sufferer. I help people just like you and me all the time. I will give you my full story later, but I have dedicated my life to doing three things: 1) bringing awareness to the epidemic that is migraine disease, 2) helping those suffering from life-altering migraines achieve a life without them, and 3) bringing awareness to this possibility for you, or someone you know and love.

Using a little-known but extremely effective method of analysis and treatment known as upper cervical specific care, my fellow practitioners and I help migraine sufferers achieve the "impossible": a life without migraines.

Now, I know what you're thinking: "A chiropractor? I've already tried several of those, to no avail..."

Or even better, maybe you haven't. Later I will demonstrate, in a lot of detail, that what you have been receiving under the label of "chiropractic" was likely not what should be practiced in a clinical setting at all.

How do I know this? Because I see it every single day. Patients that come in and think they have been under chiropractic care, but really, they've just been seeing "chiropractors" who "unstick stuck joints" or practice under the false pretense of physical therapy, massage, acupuncture, nutrition, and so on. "Hearing the crack," however, doesn't mean you will now miraculously feel better.

I stand for a world where people who are migraine sufferers have the ability to thrive in their lives, instead of merely surviving. And I can assure you that the level of specificity, detail, and analysis in this book will open your eyes to a whole new understanding of what's possible for you through upper cervical specific care versus traditional, full-spine "chiropractic" care and other methods of intervention.

Now, let me be clear: not everyone who has migraines is a candidate for the type of care we as upper cervical practitioners provide; however, those who have been everywhere, tried everything, and found nothing that works may be good candidates. Their lives are changed. Simply put, we identify a candidate for upper cervical care via sensitive and specific testing to determine an underlying nervous system dysfunction resulting from a misalignment of the upper two bones in the neck, which they were unaware of and no one has properly checked.

In a nutshell, upper cervical care is the conservative monitoring and improvement of the central nervous system—more specifically, the brain stem—by locating when a misalignment in the upper neck is present and, therefore, a correction is needed. We also identify when a misalignment is not present and intervention is not needed or warranted. The goal is always to have patients hold a correction as long as possible so that the nervous system can function optimally for as long as possible, allowing proper health, restoration, and self-healing and regulation to occur.

So, you might be a candidate, and you might not.

In part I, the book will help to make the connection between the upper cervical spine and migraines. We will then transition into a more in-depth look at how we go about distinguishing qualified candidates from unqualified ones. In part II, I will provide you with actionable items relating to committing to the journey of getting well and removing the mental road blocks that I find occur in almost 100 percent of qualified candidates and are necessary to remove in order to achieve a head-pain-free life.

We will then wrap up the book in part III, where I will explain why so many traditional routes have failed you and dive much deeper into the exact root cause that upper cervical specific care seeks to identify and eliminate. Then, I will lay out in a step-by-step fashion how to go about finding the perfect upper cervical doctor who will know how to take care of you, has been preparing their whole life to meet you, and will provide you with a life without migraines. They are going to know exactly what you are going through, what to look for, what to address, and how to help you achieve success regarding your health.

So, my question for you is this.

Are you now curious as to whether maybe, just maybe, this could be the key to unlocking your migraines?

Have you found a little hope in a solution that you had not been aware of up to this point?

Wondering where to go from here?

Curious to hear other similar stories of success in achieving a migraine-free life via the mechanism of upper cervical care?

Want to know how to find one of these 1 to 2 percent of doctors who specialize in this little-known technique?

Need some hope, strength, empowerment, and guidance to help you achieve your goal of a life without migraines?

This book was created just for you.

Part I

UNDERSTANDING YOUR MIGRAINES

CHAPTER 1

THE CONNECTION WITH UPPER CERVICAL CARE

———

She could not miss one more single day of school. She was at the end of her rope.

One more missed day of school, and she would be expelled from the eleventh grade due to absences associated with migraines. Being migraine-free was the difference between going to prom, staying on the basketball team, passing, and going to college—and failing. It was the difference between living and dying, mentally.

At sixteen years old, Lindsey was in the fourth quarter. She was out of time-outs, there was .04 seconds left on the clock, and it was time for a Hail Mary.

Migraines had completely taken over her life.

Days spent curled up in the fetal position, with black sheets draped over the large bay windows in her room, with not so much as the ceiling fan turned on to create any noise, and with enough peppermint oil on her head to deter any spiders or ants within a twenty-five-mile radius had become her new daily routine. Excedrin, Imitrex, and half a glass of water became her new breakfast, and all she wanted was to be left alone. No talk, no touch, no help, no stimulus, no noise, no lights—just the quiet of the stale room.

"Lord, if you will just make this pain go away long enough for me to open my eyes, I will do anything you ask of me," she said in her mind, over and over again, because sleep wasn't an option either.

Even worse, all of the blood work and testing done by her doctors revealed no abnormalities. All the MRI scans by her neurologist came back "inconclusive" or "unremarkable," and none of the prescribed medications had taken the edge off of the vice grip that was smashing down on her temples for the last four days straight.

She was *sick*.

In fact, she was so sick that both of her parents' jobs were in jeopardy due to the number of missed work days to tend to her doctor's visits, tests, and day-to-day medical needs. Quite frankly, at this point, neither her mom nor dad cared. They just wanted an answer.

The entire family was being affected, and a weeklong trip to the Mayo Clinic in Minnesota all the way from Little Rock, Arkansas, was becoming more and more likely. Sometimes, I've found that the most beautiful word in the English language for those in this situation is *was*, because it means something transpired in our life that changed an outcome from being in the present to becoming a thing of the past.

Let me elaborate.

Since the age of thirteen, Lindsey had been diagnosed with and suffered from "common" migraines. But ironically, like most migraines, there *was* nothing common about them. For the past three years, they had gotten progressively worse, and medications like Excedrin, Imitrex, and Topamax were becoming as weak as wet toilet paper at taking the edge off her pain.

It was then when I met Lindsey on a cold, rainy day in November 2018, as a referral from a mutual friend of ours who had heard me speak to a local group about how my mission was to locate and help the sickest of the sick suffering from migraine headaches. I wanted to work with people who had not responded to other traditional treatments, like Lindsey. In that respect, she was a perfect fit.

As I looked over her history, I was able to find exactly what I was looking for—the thing that let me know she was in the right place.

We were able to trace the migraines all the way back to a head and neck injury she had suffered three years earlier while playing basketball in the eighth grade. A little undersized and frail, she had been trying to go up for a lay-up when another player took her feet out from under her. The back of her head and neck broke her fall. It sounded like a bowling ball hitting the hardwood floor, and it echoed throughout the gym that became so quiet you could hear a pin drop.

Three months later, the migraines started. And they hadn't left her life since. It was right then that I felt very good about my chances of being able to give Lindsey and her family their lives back.

After running very specific testing of the central nervous system called Computerized Infrared Thermography (CIT), I was able to identify that her brain stem and nervous system were under an enormous amount of pressure. I then immediately initiated a three-dimensional motion X-ray series of the upper neck and head that revealed exactly what I was looking for. A misalignment of the atlas bone (the uppermost bone in the neck) was indeed present. After having the X-ray images cleared and read by a radiologist, I gave Lindsey something that I had been preparing my whole life to give her: an upper cervical correction, to address this misaligned vertebra in her upper neck that had been choking her life for over three years.

But it wasn't just any adjustment (another word for correction). It was an adjustment with that extra something. That something that gave Lindsey her life back and changed her entire situation in the blink of an eye.

She didn't have a migraine for three months after her first correction.

She now has had only one over the last two years and is going strong.

The Hail Mary was caught in the end zone for a game-winning touchdown as time expired, and the entire team celebrated, including me—and we still celebrate to this day.

My life's purpose is to help make stories like this normal, not rare. You deserve it, and you are worth it.

MIGRAINE RELIEF THROUGH UPPER CERVICAL CARE

Now, you're probably wondering, "You mean to tell me that an adjustment to the upper bone in my neck can relieve the migraines I have suffered from for more than twenty years?"

The true answer to that is I don't know. What I do as an upper cervical specific doctor isn't the end-all, cure-all for everyone suffering from headaches and migraines—or fibromyalgia or trigeminal neuralgia, for that matter. But for those I find are qualified candidates for this type of care, it has proven to be life changing. I want to be super clear, though: not everyone who is suffering, including you, is a candidate for this type of care, but everyone suffering should be checked for the possibility.

You're probably also wondering, "Why have I never heard of this before? Is it something new? Some new form of chiropractic and healthcare that is only a few years old?"

Or, "I've seen a chiropractor before, who told me he adjusted me, so this can't be my problem."

I seek to answer all of these concerns, and so much more, for you as we progress through the book to help you to achieve the pain-free life you're desperately searching for.

THE MARKET-TO-MESSAGE MISMATCH

Every day, people search for "all-natural migraine relief" on Google, Yelp, their personal Facebook pages, and everywhere else like their life depended on it! And likewise, there are upper cervical doctors looking to locate, identify, and help this same demographic of people.

What's crazy is that up to this point, the match made in heaven has not been happening!

Now, this is occurring for several reasons. I will address many of them in later chapters, but I want to specifically address one. I believe misinformation is the number one reason for the market-to-message mismatch regarding upper cervical doctors' great results with certain candidates.

We live in an era when information is readily available to us. Via the internet, social media, and digital print, virtually anybody—regardless of credibility or validity—can put things "out there" for people to consume.

And much of it, we are finding, is false—"fake news," if you will.

Well, chiropractic, and more specifically upper cervical care, is not immune to this phenomenon. In fact, I believe it is one of the least talked about methods of intervention for headache and migraine sufferers.

Why?

There are many reasons, but one of them is that many people, including chiropractors, don't know that upper cervical specific care was developed at the same time chiropractic was being developed in the early 1900s. It's important that I expand on that topic a bit further, and I think you'll find it interesting.

B.J. PALMER AND THE ADVENT OF CHIROPRACTIC

In the early 1920s, B.J. Palmer, the developer of chiropractic, was witnessing extremely good results with the most complex cases that didn't respond to traditional medicinal routes—conditions like kidney and liver disease, chronic spinal pain, complex digestive disorders, and even migraine headaches and seizures!

Palmer's results were so respected nationally that he was even receiving referrals from doctors at the Mayo Clinic in Minnesota! He had a research clinic in Davenport, Iowa, where people from all over the world would come to receive upper cervical specific care—the very same care most providers still offer today, but with more potent and advanced technology at our disposal.

But we didn't have science, technology, or research yet to validate why he was seeing such unbelievable results via the gateway to healing that is the upper cervical complex of the neck and nervous system.

So, it wasn't widely talked about and was often chalked up to "voodoo medicine," "witchcraft," or "nonscientific placebo effect."

Furthermore, when B.J. Palmer died in the early 1960s and chiropractors gained third-party insurance reimbursement rights (which I will discuss in depth in a later chapter), the upper cervical work, its marketing, and its further development more or less died with him.

However, a very small percentage of chiropractic practitioners still carry this work on today. Frankly, I believe less than 2 percent of practicing chiropractors are trained and practice upper cervical specific care exclusively. Sure, there are some who claim to be "upper cervical doctors" and dabble in the upper neck a little bit, before moving down and adjusting other vertebrae also. But when I say upper cervical specific care, I mean doctors who know everything there is to know about the upper two bones in the neck and their relationship to the brain stem—and who focus on ONLY that.

So, awareness of this option is low among migraine sufferers because we didn't have the scientific validation or research to explain the unbelievable results for a long period of time after its inception, and we also have a very small percentage of doctors who truly know how to analyze the upper cervical spine in this way.

But we do have the validation now.

The science, research, and technology now at our disposal is catching up to the philosophy that we as upper cervical care providers have witnessed and believed since Dr. Palmer discovered it in the early 1920s.

HOW A SIMPLE UPPER NECK MISALIGNMENT CAN CAUSE MIGRAINES

The brain stem facilitates the healing power of the body as the "Houston Control Center" of the nervous system, regulating all aspects of function within the human body.

It is also the major highway system of travel for all the blood supply traveling from the heart to the brain, which must pass through a very small hole, four to eight centimeters in circumference, inside the upper bone in the neck (the atlas).

Also, the major drainage system for all cerebrospinal fluid traveling to and from the brain into the spinal column drains through this very same hole in the middle of the upper bone in the neck.

A misalignment of this bone can affect all three of these crucial elements to health and equilibrium within the body. When left uncorrected long enough, it can begin to produce a warning sign going off in your upper neck and head in the form of a headache, or severe migraine, depending on the level of dysfunction.

There are more and more studies coming out by medical professionals and other researchers validating that the upper two bones of the neck and the brain stem could be HUGE contributors to the development of long-term migraines. I have included some of those references here (https://link.springer.com/article/10.1007/s11916-003-0036-y), and refer to them again in chapter 7. If this is the root cause, medications cannot, and often will not, produce a long-term benefit to migraine patients, because these medications and other medical interventions *cannot* fix this upper neck misalignment.

ARE CHIROPRACTORS QUACKS?

Most people are not aware that there is specialization within chiropractic, where all the emphasis is on analyzing, addressing, and treating the top two vertebrae of the neck only. Nothing more, and nothing less. Most people are only familiar with chiropractors who "adjust" an individual's entire spine. I will address the reason I put "adjust" in quotations later.

Furthermore, most people are not aware that this specialization called upper cervical specific care sees as high as an 80 percent success rate in eliminating migraine headaches without the use of drugs, surgeries, pills, potions, or lotions.

Now, you may be thinking, "But Dr. Grant, I've been to several chiropractors before...even ones who told me that they 'adjusted' and 'addressed' the upper two bones of the neck, and it didn't help me." Or, you might have always heard chiropractors were "quacks," "not real doctors," and most definitely not people who could help you.

And, to some extent, I would agree with you. Just like in any other profession, there are always a couple of bad apples that spoil the bushel. Some chiropractors are "quacks" and are not practicing chiropractic in the way that it was created and designed to be practiced. They don't take proper imaging that identifies a proper chiropractic candidate. They don't take imaging pre- and post-adjustment to ensure that an adjustment was indeed achieved. I also have come across some chiropractors who don't even X-ray their patients, chiropractors who blindly "adjust" patients every single visit, and the list goes on.

Similarly, there are bad lawyers, bad financial advisers, bad medical doctors, and bad massage therapists. This problem is in every service-based industry, and no profession is immune to it.

There is a uniqueness to certain upper cervical practitioners, and the results speak for themselves. However, you have to know exactly which provider is right for you in eliminating your migraines; there are certain key questions, and key things to be aware of, which I will certainly cover and bring to your attention in more depth in chapter 8.

But the first thing a practitioner should always do is assess whether you're a candidate for upper cervical care, or even chiropractic care in general.

WHAT MAKES SOMEONE A CANDIDATE FOR UPPER CERVICAL CARE?

Now, I'm not saying that upper cervical care is the answer for everybody and every condition. It is most certainly not the be-all and end-all for everybody suffering from migraines. However, in a certain population, especially those who have been exposed at some point in their life to head trauma, I have found that this can be extremely effective for candidates for this type of care. Things such as car wrecks, blows to the head, falls, sporting accidents, concussions, and traumatic brain injuries, just to name a few, can cause the underlying issue that predisposes a person to migraine headaches and makes them a candidate for upper cervical intervention.

Furthermore, those who have tried every procedure possible, and found few to no results, have much higher chances of being a candidate. Chapter 3 will cover in more detail what the computerized thermographic scan looks for specifically, but in short, we use this technology to identify an underlying central nervous system problem that warrants further investigation into the integrity of the upper two bones of the neck that house the brain stem. Essentially, the type of testing we utilize is the gold standard in determining someone as a candidate for upper cervical care. A doctor just assuming the correct course of action based on what you tell them or what they "feel" is, quite honestly, what has created such a discrepancy in competent providers versus incompetent ones.

WHY IS UPPER CERVICAL CARE SO LITTLE KNOWN?

There are three main reasons upper cervical care is little-known, unique, seldom talked about, and not something a large percentage of the world is aware of currently.

The first, which I touched on briefly earlier, is that there are not very many exclusively upper cervical practitioners in the world. We are a rarity. In fact, less than 5 percent of all chiropractors in the world are exclusively upper cervical providers, meaning all they adjust or analyze is the upper cervical area, NOTHING else. This reason is largely tied to the second one.

The second reason is because the work is extremely difficult, and consequently, rarely found in most chiropractic college curriculums. Most chiropractic colleges teach the traditional full-spine approaches, instrument-adjusting methods, methods of physical therapy, and rehab methods, but only in a handful of schools in the US will you find upper cervical analysis taught at all. The reason for this is puzzling, and still something I struggle to understand daily, but it's nonetheless true. Much like in the medical community, the more specialized the field of study, the fewer the number of doctors who complete it.

As an upper cervical doctor myself, I can attest to the fact that the work is very difficult, which is why it is seldom used by practicing chiropractors—and why you probably didn't know about its existence. It is difficult because it is the most important and delicate part of your spine, brain stem, and nervous system, and it involves a very tough analysis requiring a lot of science and technology. It is *much* more than just the analysis of "feeling the spine and crunching it." It is much more than just rubbing a cream on someone's back, throwing them on a massage table, or hooking them up to electrodes and machines. Upper cervical docs are concerned with real, objective, and tangible data, science, and technology to validate when, if, and how the patient is improving in a way that is measurable and reproducible.

You may have heard of the story of Christopher Reeve, who played Superman: he became a quadriplegic after being involved in an accident while riding a horse and tragically suffering a neck injury. But what most people don't know is that he only broke the uppermost bone in his neck (the atlas). This particular injury left him unable to feel sensation in any part of his body, and he lost the ability to move his limbs, breathe on his own, eat on his own, or perform many other vital functions to his health. His experience serves as a reminder of how delicate and important that area of your body is to your overall health and well-being.

So, while that bone, in your case, may not be fractured, if it is slightly misaligned, you might be suffering from less drastic yet still significant health challenges, such as migraines. Therefore, an expert in only that area is necessary but also difficult to find. Treating injuries to that bone, such as the one that ended Christopher Reeve's life, allows us as upper cervical doctors the ability to *save* lives every single day, *if* you know how to apply this technique appropriately. (I'll reference this story again later.) But it's difficult to obtain the rigorous training required to go about taking care of this area, and it requires a highly analytical and outside-the-box type of mind that, quite frankly, few chiropractors possess.

The third and final reason comes down to two words: insurance reimbursement. In the early 1960s, chiropractors began to demand that health insurance companies offer benefits to reimburse chiropractic services. In the beginning, this seemed at a basic level like a great idea. However, as it rolled out and became a reality, the way that the reimbursement system was created inherently pointed more and more new doctors to the traditional, full-spine approach. And here is how...

The way that reimbursement works for chiropractic services is the doctor gets paid based on how many "regions" of the spine are adjusted. Yes, you heard that right. For these purposes, there are five regions of the spine. The neck (cervical) region, thoracic (mid-back) region, lumbar (lower back) region, the sacral (pelvic) region, and the extremities (arms, hands, legs, etc.). If the insurance company pays fifteen dollars per region, as an example, how many regions of the spine do you think a chiropractor wants to adjust?

All of them.

They want to make as much money as they possibly can off that one patient visit. It's human nature. This situation made it wise and more economically advantageous for chiropractors to take an "entire spine" approach, and it diluted the upper cervical specific work, which only addresses one of the five regions of the spine.

Now, I'm not saying that all chiropractors are money-hungry pigs, but I am saying the financial gain one can make by choosing to practice the full-spine approach versus a specific approach that would make me 80 percent less under the insurance model became an easy choice for those who practiced during what is now referred to as "the Mercedes '80s." Frankly, the insurance game washed out the desire for any chiropractors to practice in a specialized environment; they felt like it was a bad business move. It is still a concern and makes practicing in this way a very bold, yet rewarding, move. But it is a major reason why it is little known and little utilized.

MY LIFE'S PURPOSE

I, like you, was also a migraine sufferer. I still to this day get checked regularly and continue to battle headaches and migraines. I've known what it's like to live life riddled with migraines, but I also know what it looks like to live a life without them.

As a collegiate athlete playing baseball and pursuing a degree in biology at the age of twenty, I found myself performing at a lower and lower level of productivity, both on and off the field, due to recurring head pain.

Upper cervical care truly saved me and gave me my life back. So, I have dedicated my life to helping people in the very same situation regain a life on their terms through the facilitation of upper cervical specific chiropractic. I had an epiphany one day when I literally thought, "It is wrong of me not to spread this message to the world, that a life without migraines can be achieved for those who truly can benefit."

I asked myself, "Grant, if you had a cure for cancer, would you share it with the world and the people who need to hear it? Or would you just keep it to yourself?"

Seriously, imagine if you stumbled across a hidden cave in the mountains of Switzerland with mysterious plants that, if eaten, completely demolished cancer cells and had the potential to save thousands of lives. If you kept it to yourself and didn't share it with the world, most would agree it would be *unethical of you*.

You would have a moral obligation to share the information to better humanity, and to *not* share that information would make you an evil and selfish person. Wouldn't you agree?

I, too, feel like I have a moral obligation to share information with the world—and you.

You see, the number one thing that I hear from every single migraine patient I have helped manage to a life free of pain is: "I have been suffering for ____ years. Why did nobody tell me this existed? Why is this not common knowledge?" or "I would have pursued this so much earlier had I known..."

So, I have dedicated my entire life's work to pursuing the dream that one day every man, woman, and child (especially migraine sufferers) will have the opportunity to experience the benefits that upper cervical care can provide in eliminating pain and suffering from people's lives—a world where "I wasn't aware" is no longer in our vocabulary.

I chose to be a chiropractor because I wanted to help save people's lives. I understood early on that since B.J. Palmer developed the profession, it was to take care of the sick and suffering, as I described in the introduction.

Notice that nowhere in there did I mention wanting to "crack people's backs."

I legitimately then, and still to this day, am only concerned with helping the sickest of the sick get well. As I went through my journey in becoming a chiropractor, I had many, many questions that went unanswered by professors, doctors, and teachers.

For instance, "How do I know this person actually needs this? How can I show this person that they, indeed, have a problem?" More importantly, "How can I show them that it is fixed or improving?"

And most importantly, "At what point is my intervention no longer necessary?"

I always thought to myself, if any of these questions are not answered for my future patients and my future self, how can I lay my head on the pillow at night knowing I commanded a fee for my services from a place of integrity?

All the methods I was being taught in school did not answer these questions for me. The approach largely relied on a very subjective "feeling" or "palpating" of the spine, and nothing was really based on *objective* or *visible* evidence. I would "feel" someone's spine for "stuck joints" while they lay on the table and would be challenged by a professor that I wasn't "feeling" the correct thing. It was frustrating to say the least, and it began to help me understand why over 90 percent of the population didn't seek out chiropractic: it didn't make sense.

For example, imagine going on a Weight Watchers diet regimen, and the weight loss coach came up, "felt" your waist, and then sent you into a rigorous eight-month program of dieting and exercise. If you returned in eight months and they only "felt" your waist again, telling you that you had done so well in losing weight, how would you feel?

You would be *pissed*. You would want real numbers to validate just how much improvement you had made! This dynamic illustrates the battle and struggle that was going on inside my head about my understanding of chiropractic being taught to me.

I needed more. Much like you, I needed answers.

I found an answer by discovering upper cervical care.

It just makes sense. Upper cervical care is the analysis, detection, and location of brain stem and nervous system pressure caused by a misaligned vertebra in the upper neck, which is disrupting the normal flow of nerve impulses traveling between the brain and the rest of the body, as well as inhibiting proper blood and cerebrospinal fluid flow traveling to and from the brain. It is not always present, and is not present in all people. But when it is, not knowing about it can be tragic, and the discovery of it is often life changing.

And yes, it is coming to fruition every single day in my clinic, The Specific Chiropractic Centers–Little Rock, as well as in our seventeen clinics around the United States and in the other clinics around the world that utilize our unique specialty within chiropractic every single day.

LISA: A MIGRAINE SUFFERER FOR TWENTY YEARS—AND WHY I WROTE THIS BOOK

Let's take Lisa, for example. Lisa presented to my office like the vast majority of patients I bring under my care do. She'd had migraine headaches for the past twenty years, at least two or three times a week. She traveled two and a half hours from a town in Arkansas called Greenwood to Little Rock looking for any semblance of hope. She was spending most of her days unable to work due to relentless, throbbing, and pulsating pain in the back of her head, traveling in behind her right eye.

The only way she could find relief was to sit with her head slightly elevated on a pillow in her bed, on her back, in complete silence and darkness. She had been taking Topamax daily as a preventative and Nortriptyline as needed. Unfortunately, both were working less and less effectively by the day, and she was beginning to worry that something was *seriously* wrong. Thank goodness, she had heard about my office through a mutual friend of ours and called to set up an appointment.

On our first encounter, she showed up with her husband (who drove her), in tears, because she'd been suffering from a weeklong headache at that point, and she couldn't even make the drive. As I was examining her, we always had to keep a trash can close by because she was nauseated and felt like she could throw up at any second. To say she was sick was an understatement. Her husband had a look in his eyes that I will never forget. It was the look of pure helplessness, and he was subconsciously telling me, "Please help us...We can't live like this anymore."

After running some CIT tests of her nervous system, I could tell that she was a candidate, and I was definitely going to be able to help.

I gave Lisa her first atlas correction three days later, and she was even worse at that time than during our first examination encounter. The headache had now begun to move from the back of the head to the front, the temples, and both eyes. She later told me that she was in the darkest state, mentally, she had ever experienced.

I rested her for forty minutes (double the usual twenty

minutes I normally rest patients) after that first correction to ensure that her neck could hold the proper alignment for as long as possible, since she had to make the two-and-a-half-hour trek back to Greenwood. I then ran a post-scan to confirm we had indeed removed pressure to the brain stem. I sent her on her way and told her to come back for a follow-up appointment two days later.

Fast forward two days, and she returned with the news that I had hoped and prayed for. She stated that as she was riding back home, it felt as if her head was "draining like water in the bathtub after removing the plug." She reported going home and sleeping undisturbed for nine straight hours, which she'd been unable to do for months prior due to pain.

As I continued to monitor her over the next six months, she did not have a single migraine after the initiation of her first correction. While there were a few low-grade, dull, achy headaches and some neck stiffness, she was no longer suffering.

She now lives months on end pain-free and was able to return to work as a full-time nanny and a part-time online clothing sales rep, within six months after her first correction.

But there was a moment as I discharged her from her

corrective care plan that broke my heart and was the inspiration behind my need to write this book for you.

As we were going over her progress and celebrating together the fact that her life was so much better and different, she asked me a question that I will never forget.

She said, "Dr. Grant, I have had a question in my head for the last two months that I have been dying to ask you..."

"What's that?" I said.

"I have suffered for twenty years from these migraines. They had completely taken over every aspect of my life, and I was at the breaking point. I was in such a horrible place mentally that I had crazy thoughts going on in my head that I have never told anyone about, not even my husband. Why did nobody tell me that something like this existed? What if Bobby would have never told me about you, or upper cervical?"

I paused and realized for the first time that I honestly couldn't answer her question. It broke my heart, and it hit me like a ton of bricks.

What if no one had told her? How different would her life look, and would she have been able to continue living this way?

In that moment, I realized how important it was that I write this book and bring awareness to you, and those like you, who are suffering from debilitating and life-altering headaches and migraines. So many people have no idea there is hope—that there is a place established just for you, and a doctor who understands your needs and knows how to partner with you along the way to make sure that you get the truth. True healing is possible, and you are not a lost cause. It wasn't about me or her anymore; it was about humanity.

Maybe you, like Lisa, have been everywhere and tried everything. Maybe you are someone who has constantly been met by failure at every single traditional medical and alternative treatment known to man, someone who, at all costs, must live your life looking to eliminate "triggers." You now have the awareness of what upper cervical care can potentially offer you, and I have painted a picture of what is possible.

So, as we investigate the reasons why all of these other routes proved ineffective, establish why triggers were never the problem, and see why this method proves so successful in certain candidates, I want you to know: you can find hope and comfort in the fact that, like Lisa and many others have discovered, a life without migraines *is* achievable.

CHAPTER 2

TRIGGERS ARE 100 PERCENT MYTH

———

Wine. Weather. Peppermint. Sound. Cheese. Your cycle. Stress. Bright lights.

They all suck.

At some point in your life, you have probably looked at some or all of these as the "trigger" for your migraines. They are just some of the more common ones that I have identified in working with hundreds of migraine sufferers. You may have even been able to locate or identify some that I did not list or are less common. Nevertheless, you have probably become accustomed to living your life by avoiding your "triggers" at all costs.

You may even feel forced to give up things you love, the way Angie did.

ANGIE: THE WOMAN WHO COULDN'T DRINK WINE

Angie showed up in my office on a rainy Thursday morning to be evaluated with one goal in mind: "I want to be able to drink wine and not wake up with a migraine!"

"I know that wine is my trigger," she said, "and I had to just give it up altogether because it was completely ruining my life. But what I have noticed is that I am getting migraines even when I don't drink wine now. So now I can't drink wine, which I love, and I still get migraines."

If you are like Angie and wine is your thing, then you can relate to how bad her life had sucked up to the point when I first met her. There is nothing worse than having to completely give up something that you thoroughly enjoy in life because you have told yourself that it "has to go."

As I began to ask her a few more questions related to her health history and "triggers," I began to bring to her attention that she felt like weather was a trigger. So was bright light—and loud sounds, such as music in the car or her kids playing loudly in the house. And stress! *Literally everything* was a trigger!

"Oh my gosh, I never realized I had so many triggers," she said. "I just always thought it was wine mostly, because it is my favorite out of them all!"

Have you ever noticed that your main trigger for sparking a migraine is usually always the one thing you love most?!

Maybe, like Angie, you love wine and cheese, but you have to avoid them all costs because within four hours of indulging, a horrible two-day migraine crisis is sure to hit. Then, it will have you popping Imitrex and Nortriptyline out of a PEZ dispenser.

But it's never the thing that you hate or dislike, or the one that's easy to give up, that seems to be the one trigger with a vice grip on your forehead.

Here is what I have come to find out in helping hundreds achieve a life without migraines:

Triggers are 100 percent myth!

Yes, I said it: they are a myth! A 100 percent myth! A hoax!

They are something that you have come to blame your migraines on because nobody has been able to give you an answer, any guidance, or direction regarding what is truly causing your migraines to keep showing up.

THE BRAIN WANTS AN EXCUSE

See, when you are in chronic pain for as long as you have

been in pain, and you're suffering, the brain forces you to provide yourself an answer or a reason. When you go from provider to provider, and bounce from treatment to treatment, you can't live with suffering without some sort of reason in your head, or it drives you to insanity!

The trigger is the easiest thing for migraine sufferers to convince themselves is the reason for why they keep suffering repeatedly. But if triggers really were what caused migraines, wouldn't everybody who suffers from migraines all have the same triggers? The idea is a cop-out, an excuse, and an answer that your brain must have in order for you to continue to live a somewhat motivated life.

Now, there definitely is something to triggers, as far as the validity and merit in us identifying what you feel like causes a migraine to show up more often.

Think of it this way: when you have a problem with the upper two bones in the neck that is pressuring and creating stress on the brain stem, that situation is the starting of a roaring fire. Things like "triggers" are like pouring gasoline on top of the already roaring fire.

Do you ever feel like you have a dull, achy headache that is there for three to four solid days sometimes that is just creeping in the background of your head? You wake up with it, you go to bed with it, and it just sits with you for days on end. Then all of the sudden, out of nowhere, it creeps up and turns into a full-blown migraine—almost like the ticking of a time bomb just waiting to go off, and there is no way for you to disarm it.

That three-day, low-grade, dull, achy headache was a siren going off, created by your brain not getting a sufficient amount of blood. An enormous amount of pressure in the head backs up because the cerebrospinal fluid surrounding the brain that drains down into the spinal column is not draining appropriately. This is what has the fire started, and then when the weather, smells, stress, sounds, and other factors come around every so often, they pour on the gas—sending you into a dark room, and into the medicine cabinet, begging for help.

For example, in Angie's case, she felt like wine, cheese, and loud noises—such as when her kids were home on spring break and turning her house into a gymnasium—were definitely "triggering" her into migraine episodes.

Identifying this information early on is *crucial* in establishing your blueprint, but it is NOT the reason you continue to suffer. And identifying triggers alone will not provide you with the pain-free life you are looking for.

YOU ARE BIGGER THAN YOUR TRIGGER

Think about this: people's bodies all over the world heal every single day from horrible things such as broken bones, cancer, influenza, and infections; your body is literally covered with bacteria 100 percent of your life, which could be a trigger for sickness every day of your life, but it isn't. Why? It's because you are much bigger, stronger, and more resilient than some trigger that you decided has taken over your life and left it so desolate. Your body is amazing at healing itself and providing you with a life without pain. No weather front, wine, or stress is too big for it to overcome, so I want you to stop right now and say this out loud or in your head—no, I'm not kidding—literally say this to yourself, as it is part of the healing process:

"I am stronger than my trigger. My trigger does not define me or my life."

Once you have said that, you have now spoken it into existence, and we can expect it to come to fruition. Remember, your brain does not know the difference between perception and reality—in other words, what you perceive to be true and what is actually true. Your brain cannot distinguish the difference between the two.

YOU CAN'T REMOVE ALL "TRIGGERS"

Here's why trying to eliminate triggers is not the wise

long-term solution to achieving a pain-free life. Unless you are living in a hyperbaric chamber, a bubble, or on the moon, eliminating all triggers is 1,000 percent impossible.

If bad weather is a "trigger" for you, think about it: how are you going to live a life avoiding the weather? You can't! Or let's say that stress is a trigger for you; how are you going to avoid stress your entire life? Gravity is a stress that your body is encountering twenty-four hours a day—you cannot run from all stresses!

You get the point. Eliminating all triggers is impossible, and doing so can't be the solution we rely on to develop a long-term strategy for knocking migraines out—not reducing them a little, but knocking them out!

Instead of trying to control the variable of external triggers, we need to focus all of our efforts on dialing in the underlying factor predisposing you to that "trigger." Locating the "root cause" is always most effective, and not doing so is what causes the trigger to continue to show up more often, and with a greater punch.

I have found in a large number of people that when we locate the underlying nervous system and brain stem pressure resulting from a misalignment of the atlas bone in the upper neck, and we correct that underlying issue, not only does head pain disappear—so do the triggers!

Angie, whom I mentioned earlier, was also able to overcome her triggers and eliminate her migraines. Identifying the exact goal that will drastically change your life as it relates to your migraines is one of the most important steps early in the process. We will work extensively in chapter 4 on helping you identify your goals! For example, Angie's goal was to be able to have wine at dinner, without it causing a migraine. After we were able to identify her as a candidate for care in our office, she has now gone six months without a migraine, even after drinking red wine!

For more than six years after suffering a car accident, during she suffered a whiplash-type injury to her neck, Angie could not drink red wine without getting a migraine the next day. While stress seemed to be a huge trigger for her, which seemed to increase her red wine intake, she was also suffering through life with more migraines and less wine. I'll never forget the first time she came into the office to be checked (which we will discuss later), and she said, "I was able to drink a Silver Oak Cabernet last night, half a bottle with my husband, and I did not get a migraine!"

Again, notice the recognition of her goal when it was met!

Now, she can live her life with her dearest of red wines with no problem. However, her case was a little unique. In the first couple of months, we noticed that while she could drink wine and it no longer gave her migraines, her kids being home over the summer still caused some head pain.

So, we were able to put some meditative exercises and yoga sessions in place that, along with care in our office, eliminated her head pain completely within a six-month period.

EMILY: CONTROLLED BY THE WEATHER

Emily is a patient I have managed over the last year or so, and she has had maybe one migraine since her first correction. When she first came in, she stated that her migraines seemed to become more present and severe when rain and thunderstorms were in the area. This is a super common one I encounter with a lot of my patients. Her life was literally planned and lived around the weather report. If there was any chance of severe weather over the weekend, she could not make any plans because she knew they would be canceled due to her getting a migraine. Sounds familiar for some of you, right?!

I explained to her that life is not meant to be lived that way, constantly having to dodge the weather; in fact, it is impossible!

After locating the problem in her upper neck and establishing her as a candidate, we started her under care, and she did fabulously. Like I mentioned before, she has had only one migraine over the last year. How much different does your life look with only one migraine over the next year?

However, for her, the win was when she came in during the first month of care ecstatic! She came in one morning, with a huge smile on her face, and stated, "This weekend was the first time in a long as I can remember, where a storm came through and I did not get a migraine. The weather didn't put me down!"

Emily's goal was obvious: she didn't want to have to wake up every day and plan around what the weather was going to do.

That focus is so incredibly important; had we not established her goal on the front end, it could have gone by, and we never would have gotten to appreciate it! But when we know what our wish is and then it comes to fruition, we get to celebrate it and prime our brain for some sort of reward. Rewarding programs our brain to continue making positive strides toward not only a pain-free life but also a healthier life in general.

More importantly for Emily, for the first time, she

realized that the weather was not actually causing her migraines. She no longer had to plan her life around bad weather. This was life changing not only for her but also for her entire family. It was now possible for her to attend her son's baseball tournaments over the weekend, go camping, go shopping, and take trips—all without first having to consult her local weatherman.

ONE SIZE DOESN'T FIT ALL

The point I am trying to make is that each person is a unique case. Any provider who approaches migraine cases with a one-size-fits-all approach very often fails. One pill that eliminates all migraines, one therapy session, one remedy—these approaches do not usually prove effective. Emily's case is different from Angie's case, which is different from Lindsey's case. While I usually look for the underlying root cause, which in all of these cases is in the upper neck and the nervous system, we also need to address the other "triggers" in each individual person's case. Those can be the difference in short-term *and* long-term relief!

So, identifying the trigger is part of the plan in getting you pain-free, absolutely, but it is most definitely only a small piece of the puzzle.

However, the overarching theme and point I am trying to

make is it's a myth that triggers cause your migraines—and a terrible strategy for achieving a long-term pain-free life. It simply is not true, and I think you would agree with me that to this point, avoiding triggers has not been successful in eliminating your migraines long-term. When you were saying to yourself, "There has got to be something else going on," you were right.

Also, think about this: if triggers truly were the cause and the same in everybody, wouldn't we have found something to eliminate them all permanently by now?

I've also often found that not only are the triggers hard to attempt to control but they also will often move around and affect you differently at different times of the year. They have a tendency to be ever so fluctuating—sound familiar?

During the summer months, brightness, sun, and heat can seem to be triggers, along with dehydration, while in the spring, pollen might seem to be the trigger.

Imagine a day when you no longer have to worry about battling a lingering headache or avoiding the landmine of a trigger.

STRESSORS VERSUS TRIGGERS

There is also a huge difference between a "stressor" and a "trigger."

A stressor is something that creates a sense of anxiety, an adrenaline rush, or a sympathetic "fight or flight" response that then can place you at a higher predisposition to certain triggers. For example, a lot of migraine sufferers I work with don't realize that their work or environment is an everyday stressor, one that has them anxious and on edge every single day, which presents a playground that triggers love to come play in. Another prevalent stressor is people's diets. Drinking large amounts of caffeine with sugar, sweeteners with aspartame, or other additives is a daily stressor many people place on themselves through their morning coffee.

Once primed by this stressor and then exposed to any type of stress in your home or work environment, when you encounter a known "trigger" like bad weather, it can suddenly leave you in pain and dysfunction for the next two days, as you just try to survive the work week.

In chapter 3, I will address some of the most effective ways I have found for eliminating some of the more common stressors, but the biggest underlying stressor that nobody is aware of is the one that is residing in the upper two bones of your neck and your brain stem!

We will go into an enormous amount of detail on this very little-known stressor in a later chapter as well, but I want to set the stage now. I have found that when the body is placed in a state of anxiousness, stress, unease, "fight or flight" sympathetic response, or tension, the likelihood of the triggering of a migraine goes up exponentially. Most people I encounter are aware of that.

However, most people are not aware that one of the biggest and most detrimental causes of underlying anxiety, stress, and sympathetic overload is when the upper two bones of the neck misalign and place pressure on the brain stem. Now, I don't mean they are actually misaligning to the extent that the brain stem is being crushed, like a "bone on a nerve" type of model; what we are finding through research is that when this misalignment occurs, it sends an enormous amount of improper nerve signals into the brain stem and nervous system, creating a lot of pressure and noise.

I'll use an analogy. Let's say you and a friend are talking in a restaurant about a very important issue, and during the conversation, a mariachi band comes in and starts singing and playing music extremely loudly. We've all been there. Well, when your brain and body are trying to communicate via your nervous system, and there is a malfunction with the upper two bones of the neck, it creates interference like the mariachi band. Loud noise interferes with your nervous system's ability to carry out very important functions within your body—functions like hormone regulation, proper enzyme release, digestion, and so much more. It sends your body into chaos mode and initiates a "fight or flight" response of increased breathing rate, decreased blood flow, anxiety, and many other negative cascades of events—without there even being a stimulus externally, only internally, and unbeknownst to you.

I have found removing this underlying stressor, amongst others, is the key to quieting down the body. Doing so, in turn, makes most "triggers" negligible, almost like they disappear from your life. It's because the trigger was like the oasis mirage in the middle of the desert. It was never there to begin with, only invented and imagined in your own head to try to determine a cause. It was a myth all along. The key to true health and a pain-free life resides in the location of the underlying predisposition and stressor, not in the myth of a trigger.

CHAPTER 3

IDENTIFYING THE ROOT CAUSE OF YOUR HEAD PAIN

———

Sally came into my office in the summer of 2017 and had been suffering from headaches since the age of seven.

She was now fifty-five, and her headaches over the last twenty years or so had progressed into more migraine intensity, severity, and frequency. I began asking her a series of questions like I do every single patient I encounter, and the more she talked, the more skeptical I became that I had the answer. It always amazes me how much can be gathered just by human intuition if it's considered, listened to, and appreciated.

She had no history of head trauma or pain, and she hadn't really tried a lot of options, such as natural remedies or commonly known procedures to help her combat the issue. She was one of those we see all the time who have just been "dealing with it" or "bearing it."

The problem was the headaches were really starting to interfere with her life, and she had hit the point that most migraine sufferers face, which is the realization they have GOT to do something, and quick, because not doing something could have dire consequences.

After chatting with her for about fifteen minutes, I ran some preliminary testing that I do in my office with the aim of locating central nervous system pressure and abnormality in qualified candidates. My suspicions began to be confirmed. She was not an ideal candidate for upper cervical care, the problem wasn't coming from her upper neck, and she needed some guidance on where to go or what to do next. It was my job now to be her quarterback.

UPPER CERVICAL CARE ISN'T THE ONLY SOLUTION

Upper cervical care is not the *only* answer—and is not a cure-all for all migraine sufferers.

We see high numbers of positive results through upper cervical care. However, some people are candidates, and some, like Sally, are not.

Rather than trying to fit Sally into a box, I recognized the origin as underlying inflammation. I had recently done some research and found that traditional Chinese medicine doctors have for millennia prescribed turmeric, along with ginger root, in the form of a willow bark extract tea to help alleviate head pain and inflammation—long before we knew about medicines and man-made, synthetic fixes—and it has proven pretty effective in certain cases.

So, I looked up an easy recipe and shared it with Sally, telling her go give it a shot for about a month. I suggested that she take it daily, and if it didn't help, to come back and see me. In that case, we'd try another route (which would also give me another month to figure out the next logical referral for her).

About two months later, I was in the office seeing patients on a busy Monday morning, and Sally showed up unannounced. I was interested and curious to see what she was going to report back. You see, in dealing with migraine patients, sometimes it takes the perfect combination of intervention to completely solve the puzzle. The more extra ammo we can get, the better.

She said, "Dr. Grant, you're a genius. I have been drinking the turmeric tea every morning with breakfast"—which is the preferred method because turmeric can have a tendency to upset the stomach, which I learned the hard way via personal experimentation—"and I have only had one headache over the last two months. I can't believe it."

I have to admit, I was a little shocked myself but nevertheless very excited for Sally.

I have included that recipe here for you to try, if you have never given it a shot (remember that it is best taken in the morning with a meal to avoid upsetting the stomach):

> 1/2 ounce to 1 ounce of organic lemon juice
> 1 tablespoon of Himalayan rock salt
> 1 cup of distilled warm water
> 1 tablespoon of turmeric powder
> 1 tablespoon of honey

COMMON REASONS FOR HEAD PAIN

DISCLAIMER: While I assume most of you reading this have tried the majority of these easy fixes, they are worth noting for those who might not have. These ideas are so easy that they are certainly at least worth checking out! The following are some of the leading causes of headaches and migraines that a lot of people simply do not consider.

CHRONIC DEHYDRATION

I can't stress highly enough that most people walking around the earth today are chronically dehydrated. The brain, body, and nervous system are HIGHLY dependent on water and fluid balance to operate correctly. The Mayo Clinic recommends that men drink 3.7 liters per day and women drink 2.7 liters per day.* Most people I encounter realize when taking a close look that they don't drink even HALF that. So, check your fluid intake, and see if you are deficient!

CAFFEINE INTAKE

Caffeine is one of the primary substances Americans are addicted to today. More than cigarettes, street drugs, and alcohol, caffeine is a potent, addictive part of most daily routines. If you are consuming a lot of caffeine and find yourself suffering from head pain, one could be causing the other! Caffeine is also a powerful diuretic, which means it activates the kidneys and will dehydrate you at a much quicker pace. So, if you are also dehydrated, it will further dehydrate you. Ironically enough, if you are someone who doesn't drink a lot of caffeine, it has also been shown to help alleviate headaches (it's one of the major ingredients in Excedrin Migraine). So, evaluate

---

* "Water: How Much Should You Drink Every Day?" Mayo Clinic, September 6, 2017, https://www.mayoclinic.org/healthy-lifestyle/nutrition-and-healthy-eating/in-depth/water/art-20044256.

your coffee, Coke, and overall caffeine intake, and see if you are overdosing on caffeine!

ASPARTAME

Aspartame is a widely popular sugar alternative used by a ton of food and beverage companies as a sweetener. But most people don't realize it has also been shown to cause headaches in chronic, long-term consumers. So, make sure that you are not consuming on a daily basis any of the following that contain aspartame: diet sodas, sugar-free ice cream, reduced-calorie fruit juices, gum, yogurt, sugarless candy, or any other "sugar-free" foods or drinks. They're sugar-free because they substitute the aspartame for the sugar!

NIGHTTIME SCREEN TIME

Recent evidence indicates blue-light screen use, like your cellular device, at night before going to bed is linked to headaches and insomnia. Using blue-light-producing devices such as cell phones, iPads, or laptops up to an hour before going to bed, and especially when in the dark, has been shown to cause headaches. So, turn the technology off at least an hour before bed, and see if it helps you sleep more deeply and diminish your head pain!

ALCOHOL USE

While this one kind of goes hand-in-hand with dehydration, it is still worth taking a self-inventory of. If you are consuming alcohol on a daily or weekly basis, it could be toxifying your liver and body, as well as placing your body in a dehydration state all the time, which can cause headaches. So, if you know that your alcohol consumption is a bit on the high side, substitute it for water with electrolytes, rehydrate, detoxify, and see if your pain levels show positive signs.

SIDE EFFECT OF MEDICINES

Let's go back to Sally's case. Another important detail that we figured out related to Sally's case was that she was also taking a lot of naproxen and ibuprofen to try to combat her migraines, and both have long been known to have associated rebound headaches as a side effect. Once she started taking the turmeric tea, which was a natural anti-inflammatory, the need for her to keep taking naproxen and ibuprofen went down. Over time, she noticed an overall decrease in head pain to virtually no pain. So, start with a diary of all of the medications (both prescribed and over the counter) that you take on a daily and weekly basis, and do a self-audit of those medications and their associated side effects. Sometimes, there is a different generic form of the same medication that can be taken instead, without the side effects present.

It continues to amaze me how many people are led down the path of drugs or surgery so quickly in their journey to a pain-free life. Most people think they are practicing common sense, but often they are not. Drugs to treat head pain symptoms absolutely work for the most part, but they often add undesirable side effects, which can then lead down the road to more dysfunction and more medications.

WHEN UPPER CERVICAL CARE *IS* THE SOLUTION

If you have already tried all of the ideas above and are still suffering, then keep reading, because the rest of this book is dedicated to you. There are two main criteria that have to be met in order for a person to be a prime candidate for upper cervical care. First, upper cervical care can be the solution when specific testing of the central nervous system indicates neuropathophysiology is present. Neuropathophysiology is a fancy way to say nervous system interference, malfunction, or dysfunction. The first step in this two-step process is checking that box off. Secondly, imaging will assess for proper integrity or alignment of the upper two bones in the neck in relation to the skull. Once it has been established via this imaging that there is indeed a misalignment or structural shift in one or both of these bones, we can then establish with great certainty that upper cervical care is warranted and a person is a well-qualified candidate. We find most people who have tried everything to no avail are great candidates for upper cervical care, essentially because we look where no one else has!

BROOKE: FACED WITH "UNAVOIDABLE" SURGERY

In 2008, Brooke had been diagnosed with Arnold Chiari Type 1, which for those who don't know is a debilitating and life-altering condition in which the brain stem has begun to protrude or herniate down through the bottom of the skull into the upper neck through a hole, or foramen, called the foramen magnum. This literally causes bony pressure from the skull onto the brain stem that leads to dizziness, vomiting, vertigo, and neck pain as well as horrible headaches and migraines.

She had tried everything there was to try, and a neurosurgeon was now telling her it was time to go in and surgically relieve the pressure by removing a portion of her lower skull and a portion of the top bone in her neck. Such surgery can be very dangerous and highly invasive, but it is sometimes necessary for those in Brooke's situation who can no longer go on living life with so many severe migraine episodes. She was essentially bedridden and starting to lose hope of ever having a normal life again. If you or someone you know has Arnold Chiari, then you know exactly what we were up against.

Surgery always needs to be our last option, though it is sometimes warranted depending on the extent of damage done and the symptoms occurring as a result. However, I have witnessed firsthand on more than one occasion that "must have" surgeries can be avoided.

Brooke was very, very scared about having such a dramatic surgery, and through an active patient in our clinic we had the fortune of helping become free of head pain, she found out about our clinic specialty.

We ran a few central nervous system scans of Brooke to assure she was a quality candidate for the type of care we provide in the office, and fortunately, she was!

We initiated treatment within two days. Fast forward, and Brooke had now gone from having migraines every single day to having only two in the last eight months. She was able to go from taking three different migraine medications per day to only having to take one, as needed. Brooke's life had been completely transformed, and she was able to go back to her job as an information technologist for a large company here in Little Rock.

We see stories like hers all the time, and it holds lessons that are applicable to you. Brooke's pain was authentic. In other words, it wasn't being caused as a side effect, or from a stressor, or because of simple dehydration or aspartame poisoning. It was due to an authentic, organic originator of pain—something underlying that was undetected.

It's much like someone suffering from dehydration. Yes, you can take ibuprofen, and typically the head pain will go away. But the underlying, organic root cause of your chronic, continual headaches was not that the body was deficient in ibuprofen. It was that the body is deprived of water, and the brain is literally signaling that a water and fluid balance issue is causing havoc to the cells of your body, one that when left long-term can lead to serious health consequences. In that case, the organic, authentic pain generator is dehydration, and the answer to alleviating that generator is hydration.

Bringing the point home is that every provider you encounter or have encountered should have first and foremost—through a series of questions, a thorough review of systems, and a history—tried to evaluate whether your head pain is authentic and originating from somewhere in the body, or a side effect of something else occurring abnormally or being taken exogenously.

Therefore, one of the first things that a neurologist will often do in severe migraine situations is order an MRI to look for an organic origin of the head pain. This could be a tumor, an aneurysm, a cyst, or some other form of authentic cause that they know administering a medication will not alleviate.

The good and bad news is most of the people I encounter in severe, frustrating, and desperate migraine situations have had an MRI deemed "unremarkable," or "normal," and been given medications to try to manage the pain, only to add on weight gain, dizziness, fatigue, and all the other wonderful accompanying side effects.

We often find with these patients that the problem is not detected via an MRI—because the problem is not in the brain but rather in the upper neck. So, it goes undetected, undiagnosed, and untreated for years.

LANCE: MIGRAINES WERE "ALL IN HIS HEAD"

I'll never forget a guy we still treat to this day named Lance. He came to us after having been to several neurologists to seek help with his migraines. He had a history of playing football collegiately, which almost immediately makes him as an ideal candidate in our world without having to run any type of testing, due to the intense trauma football places on the alignment of the upper neck.

Lance had been having migraines with aura so severely that when he felt the aura come on, he immediately would have to leave work and go home due to the fear of not being able to drive once it came on full force. This obviously was interfering with his life tremendously, and he was now starting to develop anxiety due to the uncertain and unknown nature of when his next migraine could come on.

Lance started on the journey to a pain-free life in our office after being identified as a candidate, and after being under care for only six months, he has only had one migraine that prevented him from missing work. What was unique about Lance's case is that like many of the patients we encounter, he had several MRIs that were ordered by a neurologist and proved to be "unremarkable." He was told his migraines were psychosomatic and "all in his head."

Well, we knew it wasn't all in Lance's head—and because it wasn't in his head, it had to be in his neck!

Thank goodness it was, and thank goodness we found it!

Part II

COMMIT TO
THE JOURNEY

CHAPTER 4

BE YOUR OWN HERO—SET YOUR GOALS

———

The first step in your journey to a truly pain-free life starts in your own head, no pun intended.

I'm morally obligated to guide you on the journey to a life without head pain by asking you a simple but loaded question. It's a question I'm going to go out on a limb and say with great certainty that nobody has ever asked you before. It is a question foundational in establishing whether a pain-free life is truly achievable and in your future or not—and whether this book can actually change your life.

But you must promise to be 100 percent honest with yourself in answering it. In fact, the first step of the process starts in having a "come to Jesus" meeting with yourself, if you will, about this very vital question.

The question is this: if your life ended today (unbeknownst to you, and unexpectedly), and a movie was made about your life, would you perceive yourself as the villain or the hero in your own story?

I know what you're thinking: "That is a really weird, dark, and difficult question to answer."

For example, not proactively taking charge in your own recovery, perhaps even making excuses at times or self-sabotaging by explicitly exposing yourself to known stressors, has actively left you fighting against the hero side of yourself who has all of these goals and aspirations for your life. It's this constant internal battle between villain and hero that you have been battling for years, which in the end has left you feeling like the Joker, going around Gotham ruining everything.

Let me ask it in a little bit of a different context. Close your eyes for a moment and envision the answer to this question: what does your life look like without migraine headaches?

Say tomorrow you woke up, snapped your fingers, and no

longer had migraine headaches—they are never coming back. How different does your life look?

What would you now be able to do because you no longer suffer from migraines?

What becomes possible in your life?

Typically, I see two very prominent answers to this question when I ask it of people suffering from chronic head pain. The most common is "I have no idea." Basically, a life free of migraines is not something you have come to expect is achievable, or maybe you never even considered it realistic due to the many failed attempts or broken promises you have encountered along your life's journey thus far.

The other very common answer is "Way better than it does now" or "Unbelievable." You might even become emotional enough to cry at the thought of the possibility.

I know: I've read your mind. You probably answered that question similarly to yourself subconsciously, without me ever having met you, and it's because I work with people *just like you all the time*. And I must break the news to you that such an attitude will keep you from achieving your goal.

You have been sold a false sense of hope and a sour bill of goods so many times over that you have begun to beat yourself up over the decisions and routes you have taken so far, trying to find the "perfect formula" to becoming pain-free.

What I need for you to understand is that whether you believe or realize it or not, you have made yourself out to be the villain of the story that is *you* trying to get your life back. The key to true healing starts in realizing that it is not "all in your head." The migraine is the villain, and the decisions, choices, routes, and money spent up to this point were a valuable and much needed part of the process—a necessary evil, a blessing in disguise, an unanswered prayer.

Many just give up and decide their condition is "unique" and something they will just have to "learn to live with" and "manage." Basically, you have concluded there really is no solution remaining out there that you haven't tried. However, if you are reading this book, then I would beg to differ! You are the hero, not the villain, of your own life's story, which is still being written. Yes, you are at the breaking point, and yes, you are on the edge of giving up all hope. Maybe you have become depressed, desperate, and defeated, more and more every single day.

But you have not given up...because you found this book

and are still searching for answers. And for that, I commend you. You are probably at the point of being willing to try *anything*, if there is even the slightest chance it will work.

I'm also here to tell you almost every single person I work with in your exact situation finds hope, an answer, and a solution for getting life back. In fact, over 80 percent of the people who embark on the journey of receiving upper cervical care find success. It changes lives, and it truly is the best-kept secret in healthcare.

Now, I know you are also probably super frustrated at this point, to say the least. You can't seem to find an answer and are probably even more frustrated now that I have introduced such a seemingly easy solution, which could have helped you all along. But you have to quit beating yourself up, and you cannot possibly know what you don't know!

I know this is a novel concept, but there is a HUGE difference between someone being stupid and being ignorant. Stupidity is becoming aware of something that potentially could change your life and just blatantly choosing not to look into it further. Ignorance is never even being aware of something as an option to begin with. So, in short, the difference between stupidity and ignorance is simply awareness.

I am fairly certain most of you reading this never even knew there was a specialty within the chiropractic space to begin with, one that only focuses on the two upper-most bones of the neck, *much less* that it could potentially help with your migraines!

Let's use this example: it doesn't make me stupid that I had NO idea I could write off the depreciation of my truck that I purchased last year as a business expense because I use it to travel to work every day. I didn't have that beautiful revelation until I hired a high-quality CPA to bring *awareness* to that fact, which no longer made me ignorant. Then, I would have been *stupid* not to use that information to my advantage! But it took an expert in their respective field to bring awareness to this way of reducing my tax liability.

I, as an expert in the field of migraines, am no different!

The point is that you cannot possibly know what you don't know. I know it sounds very counterintuitive, but it is seriously true. The reason people become experts in certain fields is because they are bringing awareness and knowledge regarding a certain subject, cure, treatment, or answer that is not common knowledge to the general public.

I am here to bring you awareness of a little-known procedure that could be the answer you have been looking for. Even more importantly, you aren't stupid for choosing the interventions you have up to this point; you were just unaware. Now, if the information in this book has brought awareness to this treatment as an option for you and your life, and you choose to not explore further, well, then yes, that would now bring you out of the ignorant world.

So many times, I see people who have made themselves out to be the villain, when really you are an absolute rock star. A hero. A fighter. A winner. So much of the healing process and achieving a pain-free life for the long-term starts within your own head and your mindset. We will address this in more depth in a later chapter.

But let's go back to the original question, which is how much different would your life look if you woke up tomorrow and your migraines were gone forever?

The answer to this will inherently be different for every single person. Maybe migraines are interfering with your ability to be the mom you want to be. Or being pain-free will allow you to be more productive at work and take fewer sick days, which will result in you getting a promotion and making more money.

For some, recovery might mean being more active and

dropping the ten pounds you really want to lose, but you can't seem to stay on a solid workout routine because you get a headache every time you get in a groove. Or maybe you want to be able to make plans and stick to them, without having to pencil in a migraine that could come at any moment without warning. Like I said, each person's goal and impact will be unique.

But it is CRUCIAL that we start you down this road to a pain-free life by first identifying the *goal*. We must first put the coordinate or destination that we will achieve into the GPS! Notice I didn't say that we *might* achieve but that we *will* achieve. The goal needs to be something tangible and measurable, so you will know when you have hit it.

For example, several of the patients I described had a goal to become completely medication independent. They wanted to be able to live life without having to rely on daily medications and preventatives. The fear for someone like Lindsey at the ripe age of sixteen was she would have to take prescriptions for the rest of her life, which would add on other side effects and damage her liver and kidneys.

Of course, as a chiropractor, I don't make medication recommendations. However, as we comanaged her case with her MD, we were over time able to slowly reduce her intake and help her hit her goal! But we knew when we had hit our goal because it was something objective (measurable).

So, stop right now, and I want you to write your goal down somewhere, in the back of this book, in your journal, in your calendar, or in the notes on your iPhone—*somewhere*. Once you have manifested it into existence, we can begin the journey to making it become the reality! Remember, your brain doesn't know the difference between perception and reality. So, there are quite a few solutions you can use to help establish clearly defined goals and, more importantly, when they are met.

First, write down your goal.

By the way, while I'm here: you can NEVER revisit your goal too much. In fact, the more you revisit it, the better chance you have of achieving it. It's the law of proximity: the more closely you hold it to you, the higher the likelihood you'll attain it.

This goal should be different for everybody, because everybody's migraines are different. Don't ever let anyone tell you that all migraines are the same and have the same origin or fix; that just simply is not true.

An example goal would be to go an entire month without a migraine.

Another example for someone could be to go an entire year without a migraine.

Or maybe to become independent of all medication.

And yes, these are real, attainable, rational goals achieved in an upper cervical office setting every day, without the use of a drug, surgery, pill, potion, or lotion.

Now, the second part of this is the hardest.

I want you to write down underneath your goal all the reasons why you will not hit it. Most exercises have you write down all the things that will help you achieve it, but I want you to do the opposite.

Why?

Because we are going to reverse engineer your brain. If you know what the obstacles are ahead of time, we can avoid them!

Common examples would be not being committed to the process, time, money, skepticism, fear, etc. Whatever it is, identify it, embrace it, and let's crush it ahead of time.

There are two types of people in my upper cervical office.

Patient A gets phenomenal results. I'm talking over-the-top, life-altering results, potentially going months, or even years, without a headache or migraine at all. You will see Patient A on our testimonial page. They become a lifelong upper cervical advocate and refer every single person who mentions they get even an occasional headache to go see a local upper cervical doctor near them.

Then, there is Patient B. Don't get me wrong, Patient B still gets great results. But not the "scream it from the mountaintop" type of results that completely transform and change their life.

Of course, you will want to be Patient A, which is who everyone wants to be! Do you know what, almost 100 percent of the time, the difference between Patient A and Patient B is?

Two really big factors: commitment and discipline.

Those who truly find success in anything in life do so by setting a goal, making a commitment, and executing the necessary action steps required to achieve that goal.

A fancier word for this is discipline.

Secondly, I recommend creating a vision board. A vision board is simply a white board, cork board, or some other form of board that you can pin or place pictures, images, and other visually stimulating things on. For example, you might have a goal to one day run a 5K again, and migraines in your life have made that seem impossible. Find a picture of someone running a marathon and post it on there. Another example might be that you want to travel more; place a few pictures of places you would love to see in person—Niagara Falls, the Golden Gate Bridge, whatever it may be—and place them there to continually remind you of what life should look like for you when migraines are no longer plaguing you.

Lastly, I recommend forming an accountability group with other migraine sufferers, offering a safe environment where you can be around others who are on the same journey as yourself. This group should be a place where you can share goals, express frustrations, and possibly even vent at times, but most importantly, it should be a place where you can all celebrate wins and the achievement of goals as well! Each step of the journey is important to achieving this life you are looking for. While it may seem like creating a vision board, forming an accountability group, and setting clearly defined goals and rewards are tedious and pointless right now, when you see everything come to light in the way you want it to, you will realize each step had a small part in allowing you to receive freedom. I get it: the goals you are setting seem unachievable, and the light at the end of the tunnel might seem so far away. But taking these small, incremental steps daily will build one on the next. Now that we have set the destination into the GPS and we have a plan, let's roll!

CHAPTER 5

MIND OVER MATTER

OVERCOMING THE THREE DS

———

I want to take you back to an old story that my parents used to tell me all the time when I was a child.

It's a story you are probably familiar with, one commonly told to children to help them learn the lesson of perseverance and courage at a young age.

But I don't believe it is strictly limited to kids. In fact, I think the premise is most important to you and the pain-free life you are looking to gain, on your terms.

It's the story of the little engine that could.

It is about a steam engine that is traveling up a very steep hill and running out of steam. It's a clever metaphor for times we all face in life, when it seems like all we are ever doing is going uphill, especially regarding our health, and we are running out of steam.

As the little engine begins to run out of steam, tire, and consider giving up, it motivates itself to keep on going by chanting the phrase "I think I can, I think I can, I think I can."

Over, and over, and over, the engine repeats this until it reaches the top of the hill, where it can then take a deep breath of accomplishment, realizing it preserved and overcame feeling tired and worn out, through the power and will of the mind.

Migraine sufferers are the little engine that could. And your engine is running out of steam.

You may be one of those people I encounter daily who have been told, "It is all in your head."

Or, "I think you are just being a hypochondriac, and the pain you think you are having is not real."

Or, worst of all, "You are just going to have to learn to live with headaches. They will be something you have to manage and deal with the rest of your life."

There is absolutely nothing more disempowering than

being told you are out of options, that doctors have done all they can do for you.

I'm here to tell you if you have never explored upper cervical care as an option, you have NOT exhausted all options! In fact, the very option that you should have been led to from the beginning is right before your eyes!

If you are still actively searching for a solution and believe there has to be an answer, there has to be a solution, then you are just like the little engine that could. You are not out of steam, and I applaud you! You kept searching, you didn't give up, and you kept pushing yourself up the hill that is the life-altering condition of migraines. The internal conscience within you says, "I think I can find the answer, I think I can find the option, and I think I can overcome this…"

This mindset is THE single most important thing that will guide you to the mountaintop, allow you to achieve the lifestyle of your dreams, and fulfill your greatest goal: a pain-free life.

In 1993, when Coach Jim Valvano claimed his Arthur Ashe Courage Award at the ESPYs, he so famously said, "Don't give up. Don't ever give up." He made this speech as he was battling the cancer that would lead to his death shortly thereafter.

Overcoming what I call the Three Ds is the first step toward preparing the mind to achieve a pain-free life, because the mind is the most important part of the healing process. It can create the biggest roadblock to healing, which most people don't ever appreciate.

Every single patient I have helped navigate to a pain-free life has initially presented with the same three states of mind, which are crucially important because they are usually what motivate people to explore giving our office a call for help.

Depressed. Defeated. Desperate.

Those three words describe where new patients are mentally, almost 99 percent of the time.

You must understand that health is a mental, emotional, and physical game.

Often, if we do not remove the mental block to healing first, then the physical methods of upper cervical care will only last so long to relieve your physical agony; each relies heavily on the other.

Bruce Lipton, the famous biologist and author of the hit book *The Biology of Belief: Unleashing the Power of Consciousness, Matter & Miracles*, talks a lot about the mind's ability to control the body through the way we think. Essentially, he stresses there is most definitely a mind-over-matter phenomenon that occurs within all of us. He talks a lot about how miracles that occur within healthcare do so in those people who have the mental attitude that they WILL overcome their disease.

I don't mean to be grim, but literally, those who are battling diseases like cancer and become mentally depressed, defeated, and desperate tend to die or die sooner. Those who choose to fight, overcome, become empowered, pick a line, and drive through it at all costs tend to live or live longer.

What you think is so will happen. The brain doesn't know the difference between perception and reality. In other words, the brain cannot decipher between what you think is real and what is real. If you think about it, it is so.

You literally have the ability to trick your brain into thinking and perceiving that you are pain-free, well before you actually are.

If you mentally are depressed, defeated, and desperate, then your mind, brain, and spirit have created your reality, and there is no room for healing to occur.

You might be thinking, "Come on, Grant, I get that, but

can I trick my brain into thinking I am migraine-free before I ever am?"

The answer is yes.

But the strategy and execution are crucial.

We have to clear the mental block and interference occurring between your own two ears first, before we can begin addressing the root underlying cause that is most likely occurring in your upper neck, which we will address in a later chapter.

If you are seriously committed to becoming pain-free and willing to do whatever it takes, then you must follow these daily exercises to an absolute science and execute the perfect morning routine.

From now on, I recommend you start off every single morning with these three daily practices.

I have found that the start to a perfect and pain-free day is through carrying out a perfect morning routine. The acronym for the perfect morning is **AME:**

AFFIRMATION

You must wake up every single morning with words of

affirmation that you speak into existence to yourself, as well as the world around you.

Words of affirmation are also one of the five love languages identified by Gary Chapman that are talked about most frequently when looking to identify problems occurring within people's relationships. Whether it be a marital relationship, or just a social relationship, all human beings have a certain language that speaks to them the most and makes them feel the most appreciated.

I have found that people in chronic pain have fallen out of love with themselves. We have to begin to train your brain and body to fall in love with one another again.

So, I want you to start off every morning by making a positive, affirmative statement to yourself. Say it out loud as a declarative, write it on your bathroom mirror while you get ready, write it down somewhere—it doesn't really matter. However, what does matter is that you make it a habit to trigger your mind into a positive affirmation first thing in the morning.

Some examples of words of affirmation would be...

"I am unstoppable!"

"I am a healing machine!"

"I WILL overcome the adversity!"

"I am the provider for my family!"

Anything that starts with the phrase "I am," "I will," or "I can" is most certainly an affirmation. You fill in the blank and customize it to you. The most important thing is to set the tone in your own mind, first thing in the morning, that negativity will not be tolerated, and only positivity will be drawn into your life today. Energy flows to those who have the most of it and are the most positive. This has been proven over and over again by research and testing. Healing energy is no different.

MEDITATION

Meditation is nothing complex; however, I think until it becomes a habit, you will find it far more difficult than you first thought.

Meditation is nothing more than finding a quiet place and lying flat on your back with your feet slightly elevated and your neck supported with a pillow, preferably.

No background noise, no distractions, no TVs on, no cell phones nearby—nothing but COMPLETE silence.

You are going to start off with seven minutes and focus on

nothing but your breathing. If you need more guidance, download apps such as Headspace or some of the other guided meditation apps that are available, until you get the hang of the therapy of meditation.

It is VERY powerful when done correctly and in tandem with the rest of the morning routine exercises recommended.

I recommend starting at seven minutes and working your way up as long as you can go. I know some who can meditate for as long as thirty minutes!

Once you begin to incorporate this practice into your morning routine, you are paving the way for your mind to allow healing to occur, long before it occurs. We are putting your mind into a healing state. We are preparing it for upper cervical care to have the absolute maximum benefit that it can achieve for you! Think of it as prepping the kitchen for the big Christmas dinner cooking extravaganza that will be going down the next day! We are laying the groundwork.

EXERCISE

I honestly don't care what kind of exercise you choose, but doing SOME kind of exercise for fifteen to thirty minutes every single morning, once you have unleashed your affirmation for the day and meditated, is CRUCIAL for jump-starting the mind and body's healing mechanism.

Some examples could be a fifteen-minute walk on the treadmill, a twenty-minute walk around your neighborhood while you walk your dog, or even a fifteen-minute exercise video led by your favorite YouTube fitness instructor. It doesn't matter so long as you commit to some sort of exercise for at least fifteen minutes every morning.

The best part about establishing this morning routine, EVERY day from here forward, is that once it becomes a habit, it becomes a part of your daily life. I believe that a sense of accomplishment is one of the critical components to creating a sense of "self-love" again. Self-love in your life will help pave the way for overcoming the Three Ds that are strangling your life currently. Motivation and commitment can then reignite in your life once we have put these action items in place to allow you to fall in love with yourself again.

Like I mentioned before when discussing the love languages, migraines can leave you in a hopeless and loveless place for yourself, negatively impacting your work ethic toward regaining control of your life again. You will know you are on the right track when you find yourself in a state of "flow." Flow is the state of being where everything just seems to work out or "fall into place" again. By establishing your morning routine and setting the course for your day mentally through meditation and affirmation, each day you will find yourself in more of a state of flow, which will boost your motivation, confidence, and productivity in staying the course through your commitment to being well!

Part III

THE CASE
FOR UPPER
CERVICAL CARE

CHAPTER 6

WHY THE TRADITIONAL STANDARD HAS FAILED YOU

———

Let me take a stab here.

Imitrex, Topamax, Toradol, Nortriptyline, Botox injections, the Zōk, Zomig, essential oils, the Daith piercing, and the list goes on.

You have tried them all, and nothing has worked to alleviate the pain *long term*.

Have you ever sat back and thought to yourself, "Why have none of these things worked?"

Frustrating is an understatement. I've been there myself. I found myself, as a twenty-year-old college athlete, struggling to study, attend classes, get quality sleep, and perform at a high level as a collegiate student athlete due to recurring migraines.

It got to the point where I was beginning to think I couldn't continue operating at such a high level. I began to think the schedule and stress I was under were causing the problem. Like I said in chapter 2, I began to think it was the "trigger," and the "environment" around me, that I had to change.

Probably much like you, I felt like I was going about trying to find a long-lasting solution in all the wrong ways.

Days upon days of having to take ibuprofen, Excedrin Migraine, and Aleve were beginning to have me super concerned about my overall health and well-being, and making me feel very disempowered by the fact that at only twenty years old, it was only going to get worse as I got older.

Once I learned the abundance of head injuries I had succumbed to in high school could be the underlying problem, I found what proved to be a long-term solution that has life-altering results. I began to look at all the reasons why nothing was designed to work for the long term, only the short term at best, and why the truth had been hidden from me all along.

Why had the current standard of healthcare and traditional routes failed me?

Why had I been kept in the dark, like so many are, for so long?

Why is everything aimed at treating the short-term symptom and not the long-term, underlying cause?

As I pondered these questions, and ultimately ended up choosing to devote my life's work to spreading the truth about upper cervical care to more people, I came up with three very chilling reasons the current healthcare standard had failed me, and in turn, has probably also failed you.

THERE IS NO MONEY IN YOU BEING WELL LONG-TERM

It's no secret at all that one of the biggest industries in the world is the pharmaceutical industry. Every year, companies accumulate billions of dollars in revenue for producing drugs and other "treatments" to alleviate conditions such as headaches and migraines. But two questions always come to mind that have baffled me: if they were effective and worked in alleviating the problem long-term, then why are there so many different kinds, and why do I have to keep taking them over and over again, even daily, to get relief that lasts for hours, maybe days?

One word: money.

The need for you to purchase a bottle of Excedrin repeatedly is a great business model. Does Excedrin Migraine work? Yes. But we well know, only for a day or two, and then that head pain keeps coming back, leaving you reaching for the bottle out of your purse, yet again. If you are the owner of Excedrin, and the many others out there like it, this is *exactly* what you want. Like my business curriculum teacher used to say, a business that does not produce repeat customers is not a business for very long.

MOST "TRADITIONAL" ROUTES AIM TO TREAT A SYMPTOM, NOT ELIMINATE THE CAUSE

If the check engine light came on in your car, you very well could just put a piece of black tape over it, and the problem virtually disappears immediately; out of sight, out of mind. Now, you might be chuckling to yourself, saying nobody in their right mind would ever do that. The car engine would eventually blow up, and then it would cost way more to fix that much bigger problem. But I want you to stop and think for a second that such a cover-up is *exactly* what thousands upon thousands of Americans do every single day with regard to headaches and migraines.

The siren is going off in your head, with the presence of throbbing and pulsating pain, to signal there is a problem! The check engine light has come on, and instead of asking the question "What is causing this problem?" or thinking, "I should probably get to the root cause of this pain," most just place a black piece of tape over the head pain via an over-the-counter drug or a doctor's prescription. Every single one of these drugs and prescriptions is designed with one thing in common: plain and simple, turn the pain signal *off*.

Now, are these drugs effective at masking pain symptoms? Yes! But are they fixing the malfunction in the engine that causes the warning light to activate? No! Most people I talk with who are looking for a pain-free life, long-term, get this. However, what they don't seem to understand is that the longer and longer you simply mask a problem, the bigger and bigger the problem becomes.

How is that, you ask?

Because our brain and nervous system's biggest job is to act as a sensor, one that detects when something is wrong within the body. If something abnormal is going on within the body, the nervous system's job is to relay that information to the brain so that it can be processed. Then, an appropriate signal is sent down to correct the problem. So, two things happen that are extremely detrimental when we simply take a medication to mask a symptom. One, the siren is essentially turned off, while the underlying problem is still going on, and perhaps worsening. Second, the system becomes desensitized, which means that it will take a greater problem within the body to occur before the nervous system will detect it and elicit the pain or siren response a second, third, or fourth time. Over a long period of time, this desensitization creates that day we are all too familiar with, when the pain becomes so severe nothing works. It is because the problem over time has grown larger and larger until now the engine, our body, has become dysfunctional.

OUR CURRENT HEALTHCARE STANDARD BELIEVES PEOPLE COME WITH INSTRUCTIONS

I tell almost all the patients I choose to help in my clinic the very same statement upon initiating care: "Ms. _____, you do not come with a set of instructions. So, we are going to recommend care on a bespoke, custom basis to you, and your body over time will dictate how we modify and change our route of care based on its individual needs."

You see, every healthcare setting you have probably encountered up to this point has been based on a one-size-fits-all model. Patient presents with headaches = prescribe X medication.

Patient states medication is not effective = prescribe a stronger X medication. If the patient reports no relief, then refer to a neurologist, for extra imaging like an MRI or a CT to rule out pathology, tumor, or some other sort of pain originator. Most of the time, these findings are "unremarkable" or "inconclusive." Then, either a major medical procedure or surgery is recommended, which no person in their right mind wants unless they are in excruciating pain and must fix the problem at all costs. The process most people are currently led through is very cookie-cutter, and very checkbox. Once you have checked all the boxes, it usually becomes a daily act of balancing medications and remedies just to keep your quality of life as tolerable as possible. Who the heck wants to go through life in that kind of disempowered state of energy?

The truth of the matter is I have found people who are suffering from migraines do not all come with the same set of instructions, and they need different ingredients to develop a winning formula for a pain-free life. However, I have found that some—in fact, many—have the same underlying issue in the area of the upper neck and head that they are unaware of and don't even know to have checked, which is never brought to their attention. What's tragic is that the lack of knowledge makes all other recommendations not as effective as they would have been had the problem been removed.

For example, one of the biggest things I see early on in care with patients is that their medications that used to be ineffective, now become more effective. This, in turn, allows them to take a lower dose, and they are able to wean off the dosage to achieve the same effect (as recommended and comanaged alongside their medical doctor, of course). But this looks completely different for one person than it does the next person who walks in right behind them. The truth is if medications were effective at giving people a pain-free life, we wouldn't have so many different kinds, and they all would work for everyone, which we know is not the case.

I want to be very clear, though. I am not placing blame on the pharmaceutical industry, the current medical model, or anyone, for that matter. But what I am saying is surgeons perform surgery, medical doctors prescribe, and pharmaceutical companies mass produce drugs.

I am not assuming malicious intent; however, I am saying this model of care has proven ineffective, time and time again, for years. I do believe there is also a time and place for these types of interventions. Let's be real: when you are in pain, you want to be out of it now...I've been there.

But when pain is becoming increasingly present and severe, and medications and procedures start to come into play, looking at the root cause of the problem destined for long-term resolution *must* be at the forefront of a healthcare provider's mind. And by the way, there are many possible root causes of the pain you are experiencing chronically. We dove deep into this in chapter 3 already. But the current standard Americans receive today in the game of healthcare has failed you and I for too long, and I am proposing a new lens with which to look at giving you a life free of migraines, and many other conditions for that matter. Treatment can be far more effective and achievable if we use the gray matter between our ears a little more.

Take Krissy, for example. She presented to my office with a chief complaint of migraines that were so chronic and debilitating, she was starting to lose the ability to be a mother to her three children. They were between the ages of three and thirteen, and due to the amount of stress, loss of sleep, and exhaustion from the daily mom grind, after being told about my office by a mutual friend, she gave us a call.

Krissy's case still sticks out to me among the numerous migraine cases I have helped manage, not because of how severe or difficult it was (almost every chronic migraine case, as you well know, is always somewhat difficult and severe) but because of the way she described her treatment by her most recent neurologist. She told me that after being referred to a neurologist by her PCP, her neurologist had concluded that the migraines were "psychosomatic" and "all in her head." Basically, the message was due to the stress her children brought into her life on a day-to-day basis, migraines were just something made up in her head that forced her to rest—a figment of her imagination, a fake, a hoax.

I'll never forget the way I felt when she told me about this recent "diagnosis." I remember thinking, "What a disempowering and disingenuous thing to say to a mother of three, just trying to be the best mother she can be. What kind of prick says something like that to this sweet of a person who is suffering, and leaves with no hope AT ALL for ever being able to overcome migraines?"

And then it hit me: it was not the doctor's fault, either, any more than it was Krissy's. He was out of explanations and had none other than the one he had come up with. It must just be "all in your head."

Krissy was so hopeless at this point (and who wouldn't be after being told your migraines are fake?), I remember she asked me, "Dr. Grant, am I dying, or slowly deteriorating?"

You may have at some point through your migraine journey asked yourself the same question. Once you have found yourself at the bottom and begun to portray yourself as the villain, like we talked about earlier, and you start getting diagnoses of psychosomatic or "mind originating" migraines, you begin to wonder about your own mental and physical well-being. Depression and desperation for answers tend to become the new daily cycle of thought.

I think the greatest joy in life as a doctor is giving people hope again and the realization that you and your body were created to be great—not average, but GREAT. You are not dying, and it is not all in your head, *kind of.*

After six months of care in our office, Krissy now not only is a vibrant mother to her three kids but also resumed her job as a part-time assistant at the local library. She also volunteers at her church again on Wednesday nights as a nursery helper. Migraines no longer prevent her from accomplishing all the things she wants to on a daily basis.

As a migraine sufferer, is that not all you *really* are looking for?

I'm a man of truth. Here is the real truth: if you suffer

from migraines, chances are that they will, in some form, probably stick with you for the rest of your life. I tell patients all the time that I am not God. I can't just snap my fingers and make your migraines disappear forever.

But in qualified candidates, I *can* help make them less often, less severe, and less life-altering, to the point where you forget about them—without any side effects or extra surprises on the back end that most, if not all, of the other "traditional" alternatives provide.

You see, the real reason the current standard of traditional care has failed you (besides the three reasons previously mentioned) is it sold you a false reality.

It sold you via a commercial, a doctor, a pharmaceutical rep, a radio ad, a testimonial, or some other form of advertisement or endorsement that this ONE pill, potion, lotion, or procedure would solve all of your problems. The reality is there is no such thing. I have come to appreciate that there is no ONE thing or answer to solving the mystery of a debilitating migraine sufferer.

However, with that being said, I have been able to identify a PROCESS that in certain people proves very effective for helping minimize the damaging effects migraines have on millions of Americans yearly. I am excited to share this process with you, once we have laid the groundwork for the true growth and healing to begin.

CHAPTER 7

THE CHOKE POINT

WHY AND HOW THE UPPER NECK BONES BECOME MISALIGNED

———

Let's start with your first and only quiz in this book: if you had a small rock in your shoe, and it was causing you terrible, annoying, and relentless pain to your foot as you walked, would you...

A. Limp to try and avoid putting pressure on your foot
B. Place a cushion in your shoe to reduce the discomfort
C. Take a painkiller to stop the pain and numb the sensation
D. Take your shoe off and remove the small rock

I've hopefully done a good enough job up to this point at conveying that most of the interventions, remedies, medications, and routes you have entertained thus far on your journey toward a pain-free life are all basically like choosing A, B, or C in this multiple-choice scenario.

When proposing this basic question, you probably most likely scoffed, and said, "D...duh!"

But, realistically, things like Imitrex, Topamax, the Daith piercing, the Zōk, and all the other similar types of treatments do indeed work for the most part. I can't and won't argue that point with you. But they only work in the short term and most definitely are not addressing the underlying root cause from a longevity approach.

Yes, limping, placing a cushion in your shoe, and medicating for the small rock in your shoe will work effectively, but it's idiotic to think that any of those offers the answer long-term.

Long-term relief is the goal of upper cervical care when it comes to any condition, but especially in the case of migraine headaches.

Unfortunately, all of today's Western medicine approaches aim to have you walk out of the office, fill a prescription, take a pill, and get relief. But this leads to a recurring problem that requires a higher and higher dose, which costs more and more money—and still leaves the underlying cause unfixed.

In certain candidates, we as upper cervical chiropractic providers have found an underlying cause that is, in my opinion, the best-kept secret in healthcare. It is a misalignment of the two uppermost bones in the neck, and I want to spend this entire chapter explaining how it can wreak havoc on your life, and how, if it is found and corrected, you can literally get your life back, like we have seen in so many cases!

Bringing awareness to this highly sought-after type of care is something that saves lives.

For a moment, allow me to open your eyes to the wonderful world of upper cervical care.

Very often, I get the question, "What causes the upper bones in my neck to become misaligned?"

The overarching answer is trauma, whether it be emotional, mental, or most commonly, a physical trauma to the upper head or neck specifically. It might be a car wreck, fall, blow to the head, or injury during a sporting event. I have even seen cases that dated back to the birthing process itself, in young adolescents delivered in a labored or C-section birth.

Now, I'm not suggesting that doctors delivering babies are not competent at their job: what I am saying is that according to Harvard Medical School Professor Abraham Towbin, MD, over 80 percent of children born via C-section have upper neck trauma.*

Stop and ask yourself, "Have I had any blows to my head or neck?" and "Has anyone ever checked for proper alignment of the upper two bones in my neck, even since birth?"

If you can name at least one time when you have had a traumatic event (especially in the area of the upper head and neck), or a time where you were knocked unconscious, even for a brief moment, you could potentially be a candidate for upper cervical care.

You see, not every single person walking the earth who has migraine headaches is a candidate for upper cervical care. I discuss this in length at the end of chapter 3. In fact, there are no known statistics on how many migraine sufferers are candidates for care, but what I do know is that over 80 percent of the patients I take on see at least a 50 percent reduction in both the frequency and the severity of their migraines within the first twelve visits of care.

There are three major ways that a misalignment of the

---

* Guttman, G. "Blocked atlantal nerve syndrome in babies and infants." *Manuelle Medizine* (1987): 5–10.

upper cervical complex, consisting of the upper two bones in the neck and the brain stem, can present what I call a "triple crush" phenomenon, which I believe contributes to a large majority of our population's migraine headaches.

BLOOD FLOW DISRUPTION

A very large majority of the blood vessels traveling directly to and from the brain and the brain stem pass straight through the upper two bones in the neck. These vessels travel through small holes in the two upper bones in the neck, called *foramina*, like a water hose passing through a hole in a wooden fence.

So, a misalignment of these bones could result in a disruption of the blood traveling to and from the head. The blood carries oxygen and nutrients to the brain and brain stem, which now are becoming oxygen deprived. We know that neurons, especially in the brain, that don't get oxygen die very quickly. So, the body has a response to dilate or enlarge these vessels by causing them to open wider in an effort to deliver blood efficiently to the brain to keep it active and alive. You know that pounding in your head that just seems to feel like someone is beating on the insides of your skull with an ice pick?

The nerves attached to those vessels I was just talking

about that open up like Moses parting the Red Sea to take blood to the brain become irritated and inflamed, and they cause your head to beat in tandem with your heart. The situation also causes a pressure change within the head, which I will discuss in more depth in the next section on cerebrospinal fluid.

The bottom line is this misalignment, if present, can cause a blood flow delivery issue to the brain and is a major player in the development of migraines. I also believe that the first warning sign of oxygen deprivation to the brain is in the symptom of a headache or migraine. It is a warning siren going off when the body detects that the brain is not getting an adequate oxygen supply, and the neurons are potentially suffering.

I believe this could be a HUGE factor in why we are seeing memory issues such as dementia and Alzheimer's diagnosed at younger and younger ages, especially in women who also first were experiencing headaches or migraines.

The early sign of blood flow disruption to the head is the headache. Usually, people first take a medication to mask the symptom of head pain, all at the expense of neurons dying, which never gets resolved and could eventually lead to cognition and memory issues down the road. Because our medications are getting stronger and better at masking head pain, the notion that the neurons in the brain could be negatively affected is never checked until it is usually too late, unfortunately. I believe checking and addressing the upper cervical area early enough will not only lead to positive results in treating migraines but could potentially also help in the prevention of early-onset dementia and Alzheimer's. However, more research needs to be done in this area in order to further solidify this statement as fact.

CEREBROSPINAL FLUID BLOCKAGE

Do you realize that your brain and brain stem are basically a big ball of tofu floating around in a fluid-filled jar?

Your brain is literally just floating in a big bath of fluid called cerebrospinal fluid, and this fluid wraps around the brain, brain stem, and spinal cord, connecting all the way down to the lower back.

When a misalignment of the atlas (C1) and axis (C2) bones of the upper neck occurs, it causes not only a blood flow disruption like I mentioned earlier but also a disruption in the normal flow of cerebrospinal fluid (CSF) that is 100 percent necessary for proper brain and nervous system health, recovery, and repair. The CSF's primary job is to provide cushioning for the brain and spinal cord as they are housed in the bony skull and spinal column, but it is also responsible for circulating nutrients and chemicals that have been filtered from the blood, as well as removing waste products from the brain. It is the waste removal system from the blood, brain, and nervous system. So, a blockage of this system can lead to improper waste management and waste accumulation within the nervous system.

One of the main complaints that often accompanies most migraine sufferers is brain "fog," memory issues, or a sense of "slow thinking" and impaired cognitive function. I believe this inability of the CSF to properly eliminate waste from the blood–brain barrier is a large player in the development of not only the head pain symptoms but also the accompanying memory and focus issues.

The CSF is also what keeps the fluid pressure balance within the brain and spinal column consistent. This pressure staying stable, by not getting too high or too low in the head, is crucial to overall nervous system health. When this very same misalignment occurs and the CSF flow is disrupted, it also causes a pressure backup within the skull.

You ever have that migraine that is just pounding right behind one or both of your eyes, and the only thing that even begins to take the edge off is to keep your head as still as possible?

If you stepped on a water hose, it would cause the pressure to back up into the water spigot connected to that hose, and creating high pressure. This is much like what is happening in the area of the upper neck when the atlas and axis misalign, disrupting the normal CSF flow to the area of the brain stem and the rest of the spinal cord below. It creates a fluid balance and pressure problem that can be the "root cause" of head pain.

CENTRAL NERVOUS SYSTEM AND BRAIN STEM PRESSURE

The two bones of the upper cervical spine house the most important organ for you to exist as a viable human being: the brain stem. Very few will argue the importance of the brain stem, but just in case there are some who would like to, I will start with a simple story to sell you on this notion.

I mentioned this earlier, but it's worth visiting again. Christopher Reeve, who is best known for playing Superman, was a well-known equestrian enthusiast and loved riding horses competitively. One day while riding one of his horses, he fell directly on his head, fracturing the upper bone in his neck (the atlas). From that day forward, he became paralyzed from the head and neck down, and he lost all control of the functions in his body. He lost the ability to talk, swallow, eat, walk, or use the bathroom voluntarily.

One bone being fractured caused all of that dysfunction in his body.

While a very tragic and sad story, it can also teach us a lesson on just how important the brain stem is to your overall health and existence. While most of the patients I encounter have had a head trauma, it didn't fracture the atlas vertebra but was severe enough to misalign it.

So, while this misalignment is not severe enough to cause paralysis, it is severe enough to set off a cascade of events, some of which I have already described. However, the biggest detriment that this type of misalignment of the upper neck causes, in my opinion, is a pressure and a burden placed on the central nervous system and the brain stem.

As upper cervical doctors, we are able to detect when this type of central nervous system and brain stem malfunction is occurring, which is what we look for in identifying qualified candidates for our type of care. I say it over and over again, on a daily basis in my community: not everybody should be adjusted or taken under care in an upper cervical setting, but everyone should be checked for this type of underlying problem—especially those suffering from migraines and other neurological conditions that are not responding to traditional Western medicine approaches. We can detect this problem utilizing what is called Computerized Infrared Thermography

(CIT), which detects abnormal blood flow and, therefore, abnormal heat regulation to the skin of the entire body, more specifically the area of the head and neck.

It identifies when there is an issue with the brain-to-body communication, which is largely controlled by the brain stem. There is a large center located in the brain stem called the trigeminal nucleus, which is responsible for controlling the muscles of the face and head, as well as for modulating pain, temperature, and touch from the face and head.

In a misalignment situation, this center becomes sensitive and irritated, and it is well known for being a contributor to migraine head pain (which is why stimulating it via the Daith piercing mechanism has been known to be effective for short-term relief).

The upper cervical spine itself is also very dense and packed full of nerve fibers, small muscles, and ligaments that are highly sensitive to detect movement or pain to the head or neck. Because of this, we also know that these muscles, ligaments, and surrounding nerves become very inflamed, tender, and irritated when there is a misalignment that causes the head and neck to tilt. The position of the head is what dictates the movement and function of the rest of the mid-back, low back, and even the hips, knees, and feet.

When we have all three of these crucial aspects to health affected—blood flow, cerebrospinal flow, and nervous system flow—at what I like to call the "choke point" in the upper neck, it leads to what I describe as the "triple crush" phenomenon in the upper neck. Our job as upper cervical doctors is to detect the presence or absence of this underlying causation.

As mentioned before, this area of the upper neck is delicate and is a narrow pathway for VERY important structures to pass through. In fact, the circular hole that all these elements pass through in the upper neck on average is around three to five centimeters by four to six centimeters in length and width. This is why I refer to it as the "choke point"—because there is no disc in between these two vertebrae, which allows for it to misalign more easily. Plus, due to the effect of most head and neck injuries on this area, it is very vulnerable to creating a "choking," if you will, on these three different systems connecting the upper head and neck to the rest of the body.

We've actually seen in recent research done by Dr. Scott Rosa—who is also an upper cervical practitioner and is responsible for Jim McMahon's recovery from headaches and post-concussive syndrome—that the cerebrospinal fluid can actually be so backed up that it begins to travel in the entirely wrong direction, back up into the cranium, causing it to beat against the brain inside the skull. Functional real-time MRI and CT scanning of the brain looking at cerebrospinal fluid, and even blood flow through the jugular vein (which is the primary plumbing in the brain that drains blood out of the skull back to the heart), has shown that the jugular vein can actually be closed off. The cerebrospinal fluid can be so blocked that it causes a "back jet" of fluid in the wrong direction, which can have huge effects on brain and brain stem functionality.

Essentially, if the "choke point" in your upper neck is present, it is causing a structural, electrical, and plumbing problem in the house that is your upper neck and head. This is largely why many of the treatments aimed at addressing your pain up to this point have been mostly ineffective.

But, wait, it gets even crazier, and I hope this allows for an "AH HA" moment with regard to your frustration. You have probably had MRIs and CTs that have come back "unremarkable" or "normal," and the reason is because when practitioners look at those imaging modalities, they are NOT looking for this problem!

They are looking for lesions, tumors, cysts, or growths within the brain that could represent an organic root cause, which fortunately was not present in you!

This is also why I usually recommend someone suffering from long-term migraines receive an MRI study prior to being examined in our office. Why?

We want to first rule out any of those organic origins of head pain that we know are not good candidates for upper cervical care. For example, if there is a large cyst forming inside the skull pushing directly on the brain and meninges (outer covering of the brain and spinal cord)—and causing a pressure backup in the cerebrospinal fluid, blood flow, and nervous system—removing the cyst would be the first route of intervention necessary.

We can locate the "choke point" and remove that factor in the upper neck, but it's likely that will only have a minimal effect, due to the cyst that is still present within the cranium (skull).

The goal of taking care of any patient must be LONG-term benefit, restoration, and relief, and proper diagnosis and location of the problem is paramount.

With that being said, most of the cases that make their way into an upper cervical office have already had MRIs, CTs, and other forms of imaging that all revealed an "unremarkable" or "normal" finding, which may have even been the case with you.

The point is no two cases are the same, but what is certain is that not enough people suffering from life-altering migraines are checked for the presence of this "choke point" in the upper neck. My aim for this book is to bring awareness to this underlying cause that we are finding in a large majority of chronic migraine headache cases, because locating and removing it leads to life-altering results!

Now, you might be asking, "How do I get my upper neck, brain stem, and nervous system checked?" Or, "Is there a reliable, credible, and trustworthy upper cervical practitioner near me?" And lastly, but MOST importantly, "What do I need to look for in finding the right doctor for me?"

CHAPTER 8

HOW TO FIND YOUR PERFECT PROVIDER

———

Jennifer called my office early on a Monday morning and asked, "Would it be possible for me to set up a time to come talk to Dr. Grant about his unique approach and ask him a few questions?"

Of course, these types of consultations are always welcome in my office because it is usually the skeptical, inquisitive answer-seekers who do the best with our treatment.

Why?

A confused patient is never a lifetime patient, and one of my big passions is not only empowering people to achieve the life they deserve but also educating them on the value and small details regarding why their life has undergone such a huge change.

In other words, not only do I want my patients to become well but I also want them to know the how, the what, and the why behind their healing "miracle."

OK, so back to Jennifer. She came in the next day for a consultation, totally complimentary. I am a huge believer in such sessions because they allow us to see if we are a good fit for one another, at no risk whatsoever on either of our parts. I want to eliminate all confusion or concern.

Upon arriving in the office, she immediately pulled out a piece of paper, which clearly had an array of questions on it that she desired to ask me.

She started off by saying that she had been getting "adjusted" by another chiropractor in the same town for quite some time and was not very impressed or confident in the results.

She said she believed in everything chiropractic stood for: The body is a self-healing organism; when you get a cut, it heals. The healing mechanism in the body is facilitated through our nervous system. The job of chiropractors is to locate any obstructions or interferences to that healing mechanism caused by misaligned vertebrae in the spine, and remove them so that the body can then heal in the way it was designed to all along.

She was a believer. But her hang-up was feeling like the chiropractor she was seeing didn't do any of that. She felt like all they would do was lay her on her stomach on a table, "feel" her spine, and "crack" her back. She only experienced relief for a day or two, which caused her to have to keep going back, more and more frequently.

By the way, this experience is a VERY common one that I run into every single day, unfortunately.

She was frustrated, confused, and quite frankly on the verge of giving up on chiropractic, but like you, thank goodness, she hadn't given up yet!

So, she did her research and had developed a list of questions she thought might help her locate the right fit in a chiropractor, one who answered all the questions she had, and answered them CORRECTLY, to justify that they could, indeed, deliver everything chiropractic claims to be.

And as she was asking me each question, one by one, it hit me.

How many people out there don't know what to look for in finding the right provider?

Even worse, how many people out there suffering from

migraine headaches walk into a "chiropractic" setting and assume the practitioner must be the right one from them? Would they even be able to spot a bad one? Would most in the general public who are suffering from chronic migraines know which doctors are more apt to locate the "choke point" in the upper neck, as opposed to those who are poseurs?

That day, I realized I wanted to make it one of my missions to give people suffering from health conditions that are not responding to traditional routes, especially migraine headaches, a guide and a list of questions they could ask any chiropractor and call their bluff, or find a perfect match, which is crucial in getting the results you deserve.

I sincerely hope this list, and the process I have outlined in helping you find the perfect provider for you, will help you find the perfect fit—and ultimately the restorative healing results upper cervical care can and will provide!

You can walk into any upper cervical chiropractic setting and ask your provider this set of questions. Their answers will help you find the right provider for you. Like any other profession, there are some bad apples that spoil the whole bunch. This process of questioning will help weed out the duds and bring you a provider who is an expert at locating quality candidates for upper cervical care as it pertains to helping your migraine headaches:

Question #1: Is the upper cervical spine your ONLY emphasis?

Answer #1: Yes, the upper cervical spine is ALL we focus on.

Let me elaborate on this a little bit. The incorrect answer is "Yes, we ALSO do upper cervical..."

A provider who does ultrasound, e-stimulation, massage, active release, decompression, full-spine manipulation, flexion-distraction, nutrition, acupuncture, etc. AND upper cervical...is NOT a good fit. Upper cervical doctors trained in upper cervical specific care, with that being their ONLY emphasis, don't typically utilize other modalities. Why? Because philosophically, it goes against everything we believe to be true in our rationale. The underlying cause, the "choke point" as I illustrated earlier, is the number one issue we are looking to find and remove. If we can locate it and remove it, patients often get well, and the other means of pain modification are not necessary.

Question #2: What methods of technology do you use to locate the presence or absence of neuropathophysiology (abnormal nervous system physiology), which makes someone a candidate for upper cervical care?

Answer #2: Computerized Infrared Thermography, functional MRI, sEMG, or heart rate variability.

There may be a few more that could fall into this category as an accepted answer; however, these are the most accepted and used among upper cervical practitioners. You are safe if your practitioner uses any one of these. It is also key to ask if they use them EVERY single visit, before and after an adjustment is given. This is important, because without this type of technology used both pre- and postintervention (adjustment), how do we know whether we are affecting the neurology positively or negatively? The answer is you don't, with any confidence or objective clinical judgment. The gold standard, in my opinion, that you really want to look for is a practitioner who uses Computerized Infrared Thermography, heart rate variability, or both.

> **Question #3: Do you utilize X-ray or CBCT to determine a "listing," or misalignment, as part of your analysis of the upper cervical spine for everyone?**

> **Answer #3: Yes, we utilize X-ray or CBCT to locate the misalignment in the upper cervical spine (with small children and pregnant moms being the exception).**

Many chiropractors will try to tell you they can "feel" or "palpate" for a misalignment in the upper cervical spine, and that imaging is not necessary. And they're right, if you want subpar results based on something as subjective as "palpating" or "feeling" stuck or misaligned joints, then yes, it's not necessary. But upper cervical chiropractors and researchers have found that the more specific and accurate we can be at locating the exact degree of misalignment occurring in the upper cervical complex, the better the results. I also think that you, as a chronic migraine sufferer, would want us to be as accurate as possible when dealing with your brain stem, would you not agree?

Could you imagine your dentist "feeling" your teeth to look for a cavity? Of course, you would scoff and say that's ludicrous, but it's no different. In fact, I think it's worse when your doctor does it to your spine through muscles, soft tissues, ligaments, and fascia.

Furthermore, normally, the C1 vertebra (the atlas) translates, or slides, 3.5 millimeters to the left and right in relation to the C2 bone below it. I don't know about you, but I certainly can't with any integrity, honesty, or scientific premise make the claim that I can feel 3.5 millimeters of movement through an excess of five centimeters or more of soft tissue. Imaging modalities such as X-ray and CBCT give us incredible detail as to how these bones are shaped (which is different in everyone), how they are oriented (which is different in everyone), and which way they have misaligned (which is different in everyone).

Because of the complex nature of the delicate structures

in the upper neck, we like to gather as much information and detail as possible to locate the exact problem, and these types of imaging allow us to do that. They are a must, in my opinion.

Question #4: Do you adjust your patients every visit, or will there be visits when I don't need to be adjusted?

Answer #4: We check you every visit for the NEED to be adjusted, and we will only give you an adjustment during visits when you absolutely need one based on our nervous system indicators.

If you ask this question and the doctor looks immediately puzzled and perplexed, or doesn't know what you mean, then this practitioner may not be the best fit for you.

One of the main goals upper cervical practitioners wish to achieve as early and often as possible is to get our patients to HOLD their adjustments as long as possible. Now, if you have been in any type of chiropractic setting before, this could be a bit of an area we need to elaborate on. The goal of every single chiropractor should be to get you to hold adjustments, and therefore not have the NEED to adjust you. Chiropractors love to preach that a misalignment in the spine causes nerve irritation, pressure, and interference, which inhibits proper healing—but then in the next breath adjust you three times a week, every single time you come in. This means that your body is healing AT BEST a couple days at a time, and every single time you come in the office, you are in a state of dysfunction.

Imagine if every single time you went to the dentist, they filled a cavity. Every single time you show up, they fill a cavity in the back right molar. You go home, practice proper hygiene, brushing and flossing, and then six months later you come back and again hear that you need the back right molar filled. I don't know about you, but I would be finding a new dentist, or telling them just to yank my back right molar out because there obviously is no hope for me regarding that tooth!

To walk into a chiropractic office and WANT to be adjusted is like walking into a cardiac surgeon and WANTING a quadruple bypass. For any intervention to be necessary, there first has to be a problem. Chiropractic is no different. And in all honesty, if you are only receiving adjustments that hold in your spine properly for days at most, what is the point?!

Our goal in upper cervical is to allow your body to heal as long as we can possibly get it to, which means instrumentation to measure nervous system function like thermography and heart rate variability is a MUST because those are the tools we use to know when an adjustment is indicated and safe, and when it is not.

Question #5: How long are your corrective care plans typically in duration?

Answer #5: Anywhere between four and ten months based on each unique patient's ability to hold their correction.

There will be some variation in this duration of time due to differences in technique, philosophy, and patient outcomes. The point is you want to find a practitioner who recommends a corrective care plan long enough in duration, with the correct outcomes and indicators to verify that the problem was located and corrected for a long-term result.

It just makes sense, right?! If you have been suffering from chronic migraine headaches for, let's say, fifteen years, would you expect them to just disappear for the long term overnight, or even in a week?

In the case of surgery, like the repair of a ligament in the knee, the typical recommended recovery time is anywhere from twelve to fifteen months, depending on the person's unique ability to heal and recover.

Now, we're not talking about one ligament in the knee here; we're talking about a problem in the upper neck and nervous system that has lain dormant and undetected for potentially fifteen to twenty years! So, the notion that we could possibly find this problem and correct it in a matter of weeks would not be realistic.

Now, I think it's important to preface the way you should approach the doctor with regard to your questioning. Each doctor has their own way of handling inquiries regarding how and why they do what they do; I want to make sure you approach the clinic and doctor the right way to avoid any controversy or bad interactions.

The best way to handle looking for the right doctor for you is to simply to call the clinic and ask if it would be OK to set up a time to talk to the doctor and ask some questions about the type of care they provide in their office, to see whether or not you would be a good fit. Most doctors SHOULD be 100 percent OK with that, and if they're not, then you should move on to the next one! Any doctor not willing to explain or answer any questions you have about being a patient in their office is not very likely to be a good fit right off the bat, and that is a huge red flag!

I can imagine someone calling my office and saying, "Yes, I am interested in investigating whether or not Dr. Grant thinks he could help me with my migraine headaches, and if so, I would like to ask him some questions about his approach to upper cervical care, to see if we would be a good fit for one another."

I would most definitely love the opportunity to answer any questions or concerns they might have regarding how I go about identifying good candidates and helping those with migraine headaches. The large majority of upper cervical doctors should, too!

Something along those lines is a pretty safe way to inquire about becoming a new patient in the office of most upper cervical practitioners, and like I said before, if they are not willing to talk, then you probably want to move on to the next one in your search.

Let me be real with you: not all chiropractors are the same, and not even all "upper cervical chiropractors" are the same. Some claim to be upper cervical care providers but are nowhere close to addressing that area effectively. I'm sick and tired of patients being led into chiropractic offices without any idea what to look for, which often leads to bad outcomes and pissed-off patients—and rightly so!

Like I said before, the same can be said for dentists, accountants, lawyers, and the list goes on. Hopefully, this list of questions and the contents of this book are beginning to give you an idea of what to look out for, what to ask, and a process to find the good guys out there, ones who can help you if you are properly identified using the right set of criteria!

In my opinion, and from experience in managing thousands of migraine patients, there are TWO vital things that lead to successful outcomes and achieving a pain-free life that you are searching for.

The first is locating the perfect provider for you. This entire chapter lays out the right way to go about finding the right doctor for you, one who gets it!

The second is in setting proper expectations early and recognizing some key mistakes that a lot of migraine patients make in their corrective care process. Failing to understand these two criteria can lead to poor results and disappointment. Based on where I imagine you probably are in life right now, I simply won't stand for it! So, I have dedicated the entire next chapter to helping you set the proper expectations and giving you a heads-up regarding some mistakes that most migraine sufferers make in our offices—as well as how to avoid them.

You also might be wondering, "How do I go about finding an upper cervical provider near me?"

In today's world of social media, marketing, and googling, hopefully this shouldn't be too hard.

But if you are having difficulty, the best way to find an upper cervical doctor near you is to google "upper cervical specific chiropractor near me," or go to this website, and type in your city or ZIP code to locate the doctor nearest you: https://www.uppercervicalcare.com/.

QUESTIONS FOR FINDING THE PERFECT UPPER CERVICAL PROVIDER

- Question#1: Is the upper cervical spine your ONLY emphasis?

- Answer #1: Yes, the upper cervical spine is ALL we focus on.

- Question #2: What methods of technology do you use to locate the presence or absence of neuropathophysiology (abnormal nervous system physiology), which makes someone a candidate for upper cervical care?

- Answer #2: Computerized Infrared Thermography, functional MRI, sEMG, or heart rate variability.

- Question #3: Do you utilize X-ray or CBCT to determine a "listing," or misalignment, as part of your analysis of the upper cervical spine for everyone?

- Answer #3: Yes, we utilize X-ray or CBCT to locate the misalignment in the upper cervical spine on every patient (with small children and pregnant moms being the exception).

- Question #4: Do you adjust your patients every visit, or will there be visits when I don't need to be adjusted?

- Answer #4: We check you every visit for the NEED to be adjusted, and we will only give you an adjustment during visits when you absolutely need one based on our nervous system indicators.

- Question #5: How long are your corrective care plans typically in duration?

- Answer #5: Anywhere between four and ten months based on each patient's unique ability to hold their correction.

CHAPTER 9

REALISTIC EXPECTATIONS, MISTAKES TO AVOID, AND THE KICK YOU NEED

Hopefully at this stage in the game, you have received the three most important things you were hoping to find when you purchased this book: hope, a solution, and a plan of action.

Hope and a solution come from a method of care you more than likely had zero idea existed.

You now have a solution, a plan, and a strategy for investigating upper cervical care as the answer to finding the life you have desperately been searching for, and quite frankly, you deserve.

But in taking care of thousands of people, I've found a commonality in those who don't achieve the results they are looking for and don't reach the finish line completely. It surrounds setting expectations and anticipating and avoiding mistakes ahead of time that you will more than likely encounter.

It wouldn't be fair for an orthopedic surgeon to perform a complete knee replacement and then tell the patient they will be up and running again in one week. In my opinion, knowing what you can expect to see or experience is the key driver to achieving anything in life. In fact, I believe the number one killer of most businesses is not defining and meeting expectations for the consumer and the producer. We are not going to let that happen to you!

The more likely scenario is that the surgeon will set the expectation early that the process will involve a six- to twelve-month recovery before the knee has had enough time to heal and repair well enough for the person to return to full function.

I think you would agree it would be a HUGE mistake for that person, one week after a knee replacement, to try to get up and go for a morning jog.

Such an action would be foolish, but I have to tell you one of the biggest mistakes most patients—and even providers, for that matter—make is having unrealistic expectations. They don't always grasp potential mistakes they'll encounter along the journey *on the front end* of the recommended care plan.

Heather's story is a great example of this. She had been suffering from petit mal seizures and migraines with aura for years—so long that she no longer had the confidence to drive on her own for fear that a seizure, a migraine, or both, would set in, causing a wreck and potentially even harming other people. For some of you, your migraines might be at this point as well, and you can totally relate.

Like most migraine sufferers, she was taking multiple different "preventatives" daily, which added some fogginess to her speech and memory issues. As a result, I felt like we needed to address expectations and mistakes more often and clearly than most of my patients would need. One of the first things you *must* realize and expect when you find the right upper cervical provider is upper cervical care is a process. It most likely took a lot of time, and a long process, for your upper neck and head to develop a problem; likewise, it will take time and a process for your body to return to a high-functioning state again.

Heather had suffered from migraines for over twenty years, so I was very up front with her that it would take *at least* four to six months for us to feel confident that the problem in her neck, brain stem, and nervous system had been corrected. Your provider should be, too! It makes no sense to think a problem that has been around for over twenty years will resolve in a couple of weeks. Now, don't get me wrong. Patients under upper cervical care do see positive improvements, and potentially even become pain-free early, but I must caution you that such progress does not indicate by any means that the underlying problem is fully resolved.

It takes time for the body to heal, repair, and grow.

With Heather's case, I also cautioned her that one of the first things that she would probably experience was a lot of fatigue and low energy levels. Many patients who start under upper cervical care experience more fatigue than usual over the first month or so. You might be asking why.

One of the biggest issues that migraines can cause—especially in those who suffer from them daily, or even weekly—is inactivity. Because chronic pain and the nature of pain associated with migraines can be some of the worst there is, sufferers tend to find themselves more on the couch or in bed, and certainly not on any consistent routine of exercise.

Once you start to experience more and more pain-free days, the first thing you and your body will want to do is get up and go do stuff! You no longer feel like you have a ball and chain attached to your ankle. As your body beings to heal, it's typical to do more activities than you have in a long time—you go shopping, exercise, work longer hours, take a trip, and so on. So naturally, that transition back into a more active lifestyle can result in days of fatigue. But if this expectation is set early and appreciated before it happens, it will leave you more prepared to deal with the issue proactively when it does show up.

But wait...there is also a second reason fatigue is prevalent early on in care, when your nervous system begins to operate at a higher and higher level, which is ultimately the goal of care in an upper cervical setting. A major process in your body begins occurring better than it has in a long time.

Detoxification.

The pain medications, preventative medications, and interventions you have been exposed to, likely for years now, have left your body very toxic. Migraine medications in particular are very potent and toxic to your body. Over time, your body becomes able to rid and detoxify these medications at a higher and higher rate. Therefore, over time, medications tend to not work as well as they once did, and most doctors will continue to up the dose, more and more. This is because your body becomes better and faster at clearing the body through the kidneys, the urine, the skin, and all the detoxification processes it uses. Your body says, "It's time to get rid of this toxin as quickly as possible!"

But this process of detoxification also expends an enormous amount of energy. So, along with increasing your daily workload and your detoxification processes, it often leads to patients feeling a higher level of fatigue and energy loss early on in the process.

Let's go back to Heather. Early on, she had committed to staying the course through our six-month corrective care process. We told her up front that recovery would take time, and she would more than likely experience a myriad of changes during the first two to three months of care—namely fatigue, plus a few other common ones I will address. Two months into care, Heather was getting up early enough to fix her two kids' lunches, get them ready for school, take them to school, and be at work by 8:30 a.m. for the first time in over ten years...a huge change for her, obviously. As you progress to a pain-free life, these types of changes begin to happen, but they sometimes come at the expense of fatigue. Expect and appreciate it, and you will push through and adapt.

So, expect the process to take at least four to sixth months to notice a life-altering change, and expect fatigue or an energy level change within the first couple of months.

You also need to be aware of another huge expectation and mistake to avoid that is very common in my office. As you experience days, weeks, and even months without migraines, it is tempting to completely quit taking a lot of medications and remedies you have been taking for so long. While I know eventually that should be a long-term goal, it is one that needs to be properly managed with the help of your neurologist or primary care doctor.

Often, I get the question, "Dr. Grant, can I quit taking my Topamax?" Or fill in the blank with whatever daily medication you are taking.

The answer truly is that because you and I are not trained in medical pharmacology, the decision must be made in tandem with the professional who put you on that medication. Sometimes this choice is tricky and is met with some pushback by medical providers. However, most of the ones I have worked with have the right intentions and the same goal as you do, which is to help you receive the life-changing results you have been searching for.

It should be the goal of every healthcare provider on your team to help you become pain-free, independent, and self-sufficient. If someone is on your current team of providers does not adopt that philosophy and have your best interest at heart, then it might be time to fire them!

After being under care for about four months, Heather had gone from having migraines two to three times a week to only one in two months. She was beginning to do more and be a mom again. Her work output as a lawyer was beginning to increase, which she stated later was improving her self-esteem and self-appreciation. With the help of her neurologist, she began tapering her Topamax, Toradol, and Zomig until she was taking virtually nothing daily. She had pushed through an entire month of fatigue with the help of some all-natural teas, frequent naps, and all-natural supplementation recommended by her functional medicine doctor.

Everything has come full circle for her, and after being under care now for almost two years, we are happy to report that she is virtually migraine-free. She is one of the many we have taken care of who have had a life-changing experience, and she has referred many of her friends just like her to our office or to other upper cervical offices around the US.

However, Heather herself wanted me to pass along another expectation to keep in mind and a mistake to make sure you avoid. After completing her corrective care process, at the six-month mark, I asked her, "Now that you have gone through the process, what would you tell someone who is on day one of their journey and has just started their plan?"

Her answer was one I feel the need to share with you. She said the following:

> If others could have a window into the intensity of our pain, the level of compassion and understanding on the topic of migraines would undoubtedly grow exponentially. However, the reality is they can't because it's only something you live to understand. There is nothing worse than hearing someone say they understand our pain, when we know they really have no idea. They tell us it is all in our own head, and it drives us nuts! Each of us have different levels of pain, and different responses to different treatments and interventions, and have had many things fail us.
>
> My advice as you start your upper cervical journey is to first find the right doctor for you, that understands you are looking for a long-term solution, and not a quick fix; then, start off with hopes of having a few more good days, less pain, more function, and less foggy-headedness, and overall more good days than bad days. Then, you will see a day where you have more good days than you do bad days; then there will eventually be a day where you can't remember the last time you had a bad day, and over-the-

counter medications actually work and knock out your headaches. That is the measure and evidence of progress! Progress, and signs of it, will propel you into continuing on your plan! I haven't had a migraine in over two months now and am still to this day astonished at the amount of progress I have made in a relatively short period of time. Trust the process; this care has changed my life!

Heather highlights in these words of encouragement one of the last mistakes I want to caution you to avoid making as you start your journey.

Migraines do not define who you are, or what you can be... but they are forever going to be a part of your life. You'll always have to manage them.

What I mean by that is while we as upper cervical practitioners do see phenomenal results that dramatically decrease the frequency and severity of migraines in your life, none of us have ever seen a person live the rest of their life without a migraine. After all, we are not God!

I cannot snap my fingers and make your migraines disappear forever. You cannot have the expectation that any one intervention, even upper cervical care, will eliminate migraines forever from your life.

What I really am trying to say is you can fully expect that

if given the proper care, migraines should no longer alter, interfere, or inhibit your quality of life, but every once in a while, they will still try to come around.

For example, let's say when you start care with me, you have one migraine a week. Over the first three months of care, you only have three, so one per month—that means the frequency is down *drastically*. Now, you might be the kind of person who suffers so badly you're thinking, "I would LOVE to only have one a month!"

I get it, which brings me to the point. What is considered improvement or success to one person may not be a success or improvement to someone else. The results you receive are relative and are 100 percent customized and bespoke to you. You may be the type of migraine sufferer who has a goal to have only one migraine per month, while another person's life will be dramatically changed if they only get one per week. The goal of care is to get the migraines to a point where they no longer interfere with your ability to live life on your terms, and that can mean different things to different people.

But do not make the mistake of setting a goal to never have a migraine again because that will set you up to feel like you have fallen short, when you have actually made HUGE progress.

Success is always relative to the person. I urge you to keep this in mind and set an expectation and a goal that is fair to you—one you will be happy with, while also taking into consideration what is realistic.

Your doctor should also be able to help you in setting a realistic expectation, which should be reflected in the care plan they recommend for you and the goal the plan aims to help you achieve.

I mentioned this in a previous chapter, but the best way, in my opinion, to come up with a reasonable expectation is to ask yourself this question: if you woke up tomorrow, and you could snap your fingers, and your migraines were gone and never coming back (which is strictly hypothetical), how much different would your life look?

What, as far your quality of life is concerned, would migraines being gone allow you to do?

Could you return to working out again at the gym regularly? Would it allow you to spend more time with your kids?

Would it allow you to drink wine again, or stay up late working longer hours?

What kind of impact would it allow you to have on your

life, your family, your job, your friends?! It is important to attach your expectation and goal to something in this way because that is truly what will allow you to measure a successful outcome and feel good about the commitment and results YOU have achieved.

I want you to take a moment to identify what you are actually looking for because that is what has driven you to try all of the interventions you have tried. You are on a search for what most people desire in life, which is the ability to do what you want, when you want, with whom you want. Up to this point, migraines have stripped that freedom from you, and they don't have to any longer.

CONCLUSION

I want to end by congratulating you.

Not just because you finished an entire book (though that is a feat in and of itself today), but because you have found new hope.

You have found a solution you never even knew existed, one that I'm sure you are hoping has been the key to unlocking your problem all along. And I have news: if you are a candidate, it will be!

A moment of transparency on my part: when I was writing this book, I couldn't help but think about all of the men and women of the past whose lives were completely torn apart, half lived, of poor quality, and potentially even ended early because they couldn't find hope, due to the stranglehold headaches had on them. And nobody came to the rescue or provided an answer for them.

It's a statistic that will never be covered in the local news or national media, but I seriously believe headaches and migraines are secretly destroying the human experience daily.

So, I wrote this book with you in mind, in the hope it could save your life and the quality thereof!

So many people throughout your journey have left you disempowered and without hope.

People may have said things behind your back: "Do you think she really is in pain?" "Do you think she is making these migraines up?" "Nobody can be in pain that much." "He doesn't seem that sick."

All of these disempowering statements could leave you with the belief that this was life. So, good for you for continuing to search for your truth; my hope is that like so many others, you have found it in upper cervical care.

The truth is there is a solution out there; there must be, and there is.

So, where do you go from here? You have the knowledge, and knowledge is power. But sometimes, the first step is the hardest to take.

The first thing you should do is provide someone else in your circle with hope also!

There is so much power in the healing process by providing energy, healing, and hope to someone else. And there is power in someone going on the journey with you. Maybe a friend, significant other, or whoever you would deem as your "power circle."

Maybe tell them about this book or the process of upper cervical care that they undoubtedly, like you, were ignorant of. If they are close to you, they may have had to sit back and witness your suffering, so they should be just as intrigued to learn about it also!

Or send them my info, and I will send them a copy of the book myself!

In whatever way you see fit, provide this solution as an option to someone else and allow them a chance at gaining hope, and a new life, just like you have been yearning for. Believe me: it is empowering.

The second thing is to obviously find the provider who is right for you!

I promise—I talk to the few of us around the globe weekly (we're working daily to change this horrible shortage and train more upper cervical doctors to take care of more people), and they are waiting for your call. They are waiting to take your hand and walk with you every step of the way, to help you through the ups and downs of your journey.

Just keep in mind all of those expectations and mistakes to avoid when first starting out that I laid out in chapter 9. I believe finding the perfect provider is the single most important factor in determining how far your results can take you, but the second biggest factor is understanding, accepting, and anticipating all of the mistakes you could potentially make. Set the proper expectations BEFORE starting upper cervical care.

Go back and read through chapter 9, if you have forgotten or need a refresher on what some of those key expectations and mistakes are; it is paramount to achieving the full benefit on your way to a pain-free life.

Once you have completed this book, I actually think it is a good idea to write down two things on a piece of paper, on the notes in your phone, on the mirror, or somewhere that you will constantly be reminded.

This will take quite a bit of self-awareness, but I think it is also very important to come to terms with, when you decide to commit to getting well.

I am going to go ahead and put out into the universe what will transpire for you over the next six months to a year of your life so that we can make a public record before it happens.

You are going to follow the steps I laid out in the previous chapter to find your upper cervical doctor, to identify whether you are a candidate for care—NOW.

Not tomorrow, not in a week or so, but NOW.

Positive outcomes always favor the decisive.

Don't allow indecisiveness to creep into your life and steal what is attainable from you. Self-limiting beliefs like "It won't work for me," "It can't be that easy," or "I'm too complicated" are all vision and success killers.

Find nearby upper cervical providers now, make the call or go on the internet, make the appointment, vet the appropriate providers using the questions I gave you, and get plugged in!

Once you feel like you have found the closest and best option for you, and you have been recommended a treatment plan, the next most important step is to COMMIT.

I will go ahead and save you the suspense. If you plan

on "giving upper cervical a try for a few visits," IT WILL NOT WORK.

Yes, you may feel a little better and possibly go a couple days, weeks, or even months without head pain, but I can say from experience and with certainty that the problem is most definitely not fixed long-term. It takes time for the process to make a long-lasting correction to the neck and nervous system.

Many of you have been suffering from headaches or migraines for years, possibly decades! So, we can logically assume the problem in your upper neck, brain stem, and nervous system has probably been there equally as long, if not longer!

What do you have to lose by committing to the process and seeing it through?

The most beautiful part about upper cervical care is the only side effects are health and well-being. Because we are not injecting, adding to, or taking anything away from the body, in an inside-out approach, there are no dangerous side effects.

Some people will wrongly tell you there is a chance of harm, such as a stroke, in an upper cervical care setting. There is absolutely no evidence linking a chiropractic adjustment to a stroke event. You have a better chance of a deer walking into your living room and having dinner with you than you do of having a stroke from a chiropractic adjustment given properly.

The top five risk factors associated with stroke, in no particular order, are the following: high blood pressure, high blood pressure medications, diabetes, smoking, and heart disease. None of those include chiropractic care, and ironically enough, some of these are probably risk factors you might know you have!

But the point I am trying to make is that there is risk associated with everything. Getting in your car to drive to work every day assumes some sort of a risk of death. Getting chiropractic care is no different, but the risk associated with it is much lower than most things in life we do related to our health.

If you need a better example, just turn on the TV, and wait for the next pharmaceutical ad. The first twenty seconds will be about the benefits of the medication, while the other 75 percent of the ad will be side effects and risk factors associated with it. Yet most people still take such prescriptions anyway.

Don't let one of your reasons for not getting upper cervical care be this fear. The risk simply doesn't exist. There isn't any evidence to back up the claim that upper cervical care is not safe, with one caveat.

The reason I am so adamant about you finding the right provider is because finding the wrong one, who doesn't have thorough analysis and candidate-finding measures, CAN be a problem.

If you are not properly evaluated and analyzed for the presence or absence of this problem in the neck, on every single visit, then being "adjusted" in the wrong place, at the wrong times, can have negative effects. This is one of the main reasons I highly recommend not skipping any of the steps I have laid out in navigating your way to a pain-free life. You MUST follow the right path, and deviating from the laid-out itinerary or skipping any one step can lead to a different outcome from the one you or I want!

Finally, if there is anything I can do for you in answering any remaining questions related to your journey to being well, my door is always open, and my lines of communication are always clear for anyone wanting clarification regarding upper cervical care.

I truly believe that upper cervical care is the best-kept secret in healthcare, especially in the area of headache and migraine relief, without the use of any drugs, surgeries, potions, or lotions. I am excited for you, and I can't wait for you to experience what life will look like when you live it clear, without brain stem pressure or irritation and an adequate blood and cerebrospinal fluid flow to the brain. I have no doubt that like many other patients on a day-to-day basis, you will also experience many other health benefits that you never thought would be positive side effects.

Yes, POSITIVE side effects, not negative ones.

The only thing you will be asking yourself once you have finished your commitment and achieved the "impossible" is this: "Why is this not common knowledge, and why was I not led to this sooner?"

I hope this book provided value to you in the way of awareness, knowledge, and truth—and the truth residing in upper cervical care shall set you free!

ACKNOWLEDGMENTS

———

There are so many people I would like to acknowledge that I don't even know where to start, and I apologize in advance for those I've left out. I would first like to thank my Lord and savior, Jesus Christ, because without his unwavering love for us, none of this would have been possible.

Thank you to my wife for always being my biggest cheerleader, and the love of my life.

Thank you to my Mimi and Wayne, who have supported me in so many ways throughout my journey to becoming the man I am today and making my career possible.

Thank you to my parents for always putting family first and personally sacrificing their own health and happiness for the happiness of our family, and for always supporting me.

Thank you to my brothers—Matt, Cody, Jake, and Jeremy—for following me all over the world chasing a dream, and personally sacrificing so much to make my growth possible. I'm sorry I wasn't there more.

Thank you to Tucker Max, Maggie, Hal, Rachael, Zach, and the entire Scribe Media team for helping me get my message to the world.

Thank you to my mentors and friends Dr. Shawn Dill and Dr. Lacey Book for providing me the guidance, framework, and mindset to serve the people I was meant to serve and create the lifestyle of my dreams.

Thank you to my entire team of doctors at The Specific Chiropractic Centers around the globe for allowing an atmosphere where the standard is the standard and for putting the *care* back in healthcare.

Thank you to the chiropractic giants who came before me and had a conviction stronger than a desire to please, those who were jailed and put their lives on the line to keep chiropractic pure.

And last but certainly not least, a huge thank you to all the beautiful people I get the opportunity to serve and help at The Specific Chiropractic Centers in Little Rock, Arkansas. Your stories of perseverance and commitment are what most inspired me to take your message to the world of hope and healing for migraines and beyond. My "why" runs deep, but it starts with getting to be a small piece of your life and health transformation every day.

ABOUT THE AUTHOR

—

DR. GRANT DENNIS, who graduated cum laude from Parker University in 2016, owns and operates The Specific Chiropractic Centers in Little Rock, Arkansas. Dr. Dennis successfully started an all-cash upper cervical specific clinic, which became profitable within the first three months of being open and then grew to one hundred patient visits a week in a year's time. He currently manages over two hundred patients per week. As an Arkansas native, Dr. Dennis has a passion for bringing the highest standards of 100 percent pure chiropractic to the state where he was born and raised, while also providing a safe training ground for new young doctors to come learn how to heal the sick.

While in full-time private practice, Dr. Dennis also works as the chief operating officer for The Specific Chiropractic Centers franchise (which currently has seventeen clinics nationally) in the area of vendor relations, compliance, new clinic onboarding, systems, and acquisition, while also managing their International Outreach Program, in conjunction with The Art of the Specific. The program is a philanthropic initiative that provides chiropractic services to underserved and unregulated areas of the world, such as El Salvador, Mexico, and the Philippines.

Dr. Dennis is a co-instructor and serves on the board of The Art of the Specific, which is a knee chest and upper cervical specific training program designed to help students and doctors become masters in the art of knee chest adjusting, clinic systems, and processes as well as marketing, philosophy, neurology, thermography, and complex case management.

Dr. Dennis also serves as the vice president of the International Federation of Chiropractors and Organizations (IFCO) and chairs the Political Action and Student Committee to assist with the recruiting, retention, and mentorship of new students committed to preserving the detection and correction of vertebral subluxation, as well as aiding in the generation of political initiatives, positioning statements, and collaboration with state organizations and associations. He also serves locally on the board of several nonprofit organizations, including the Dorcas House and Nehemiah House run under the umbrella of the Union Rescue Mission in the greater Little Rock area.

Dr. Dennis is a proud regent and supporter of Sherman College of Chiropractic, as well as the Australian Spinal Research Foundation. He has presented research in the area of upper cervical specific care at the International Research and Philosophy Symposium. He is committed to supporting the cause and guarding the sacred trust left to him by the giants before him, by practicing in a principled way, becoming successful, and giving back support where it is needed to keep the profession moving forward while remaining unique and distinct.